DATE DUE

BRODART   Cat. No. 23-221

A Caring Approach in
Nursing Administration

JAN J. NYBERG

UNIVERSITY PRESS OF COLORADO

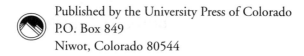
Published by the University Press of Colorado
P.O. Box 849
Niwot, Colorado 80544

The University Press of Colorado is a cooperative publishing enterprise supported, in part, by Adams State College, Colorado State University, Fort Lewis College, Mesa State College, Metropolitan State College of Denver, University of Colorado, University of Northern Colorado, University of Southern Colorado, and Western State College of Colorado.

Library of Congress Cataloging-in-Publication Data

Nyberg, Jan J., 1944–
    A caring approach in nursing administration / Jan J. Nyberg.
      p.   cm.
    Includes bibliographical references and index.
    ISBN 0-87081-478-8 (hard cover : alk. paper)
    1. Nursing services—Administration.   2. Nurse administrators.
  I. Title.
    [DNLM: 1. Nursing—organization & administration.   2. Nurse
Administrators.   WY 105 N993c 1998]
RT89.N93   1998
362.1'73'068—dc21
DNLM/DLC
for Library of Congress   97-49688
                                        CIP

This book was designed and set in
Adobe Garamond and AG Old Face
by Stephen Adams, Aspen.

10 9 8 7 6 5 4 3 2 1

ISBN 0-87081-478-8

9 780870 814785

90000

This book is dedicated to all the nurses that have passed through my life. The staff nurses who do the real work of caring, nurse managers who care for the staff and juggle a thousand responsibilities, nurse administrators who walk the fine line of supporting caring nursing within the bureaucracy, and nurse educators who taught me and allowed me to teach them.

My mentor, Dr. Eunice Blair, has been inspirational every time I have seen her. She helped me grow personally and professionally and was the reason I ever thought I could be a nurse administrator. Dr. Phyllis Schultz was my Ph.D. advisor, and she made it a mission to get me through school. With her kindness and high expectations, she brought out the best in me.

Finally, I dedicate this book to Dr. Karen Miller, who has been my closest nursing colleague and friend for fifteen years. I was her boss once and she was my boss later, but more than that, we have shared our vision and direction of nursing. After I became disabled, it was Karen who quietly insisted that my contribution to nursing was not ended. This book contains our shared views, and I thank her for helping me to get it done.

Contents

Figures

Foreword

by Jean Watson

Current mainstream books and publicity about management and administration in health care are concerned with the takeover of health care by managed-care organizations. Many provide lots of quick and externally focused answers. Many of them are economically driven, to the exclusion of humans, values, ethics, and the human spirit of all those who pass through systems as deliverers and receivers of care. On the other hand, there is a new generation of works that address new forms of administration and leadership—works that inspire and evoke foundational changes in health care and forms of organizational leadership and management. This work by Dr. Jan Nyberg is guided by a lifelong career of administration and management that is informed by deeper human dimensions of caring, and more lasting approaches to change than quick-fix, economic takeovers.

Jan Nyberg, an experienced nursing administrator, scholar, and educator, knows another way—from the inside out rather than the outside in. She brings forth her wisdom and knowledge, experiences, and insights so that others may now grasp another way to transform systems for delivery of human caring and healing. This work informs, instructs, and inspires; it invites nurse leaders and other health administrators to reach for what might be, rather than succumbing to what already is.

This work can be considered a source of healing and renewal for practicing nurses and nurse administrators. Nurses who have endured systems and styles of administration that deplete the human spirit and stifle the growth, hope, and possibilities of both people and systems can now find other options. A caring approach to nursing administration is presented that mirrors one's values, ethics, philosophy, and intention for delivering and administering human caring services.

The book's focus is on nursing administration, but the style of leadership and administration proposed is grounded in philosophy, theory, and an ethic of caring. The author translates a human caring orientation into caring at the organizational level. In each progressive step in the book, from caring theory to caring in administration, to organizational theory, to leadership styles, to the health care system as a whole, the author is guided and informed by years of administration—years when she was experienced by hundreds, if not thousands of nurses as an inspirational leader who exemplified caring in nursing administration.

Therefore, the author has successfully practiced her theory and philosophy with nurses and others throughout her career. However, do not be misled. While the background for this work comes from nursing, the foreground embraces and affects the entire health care system of management and administration. The scope of the work extends to caring and nursing economics; the search for values and ethics; research in caring and administration; organizational effectiveness and quality management; and understanding and organizing the work of nursing, concluding with the practice of nursing administration.

Jan Nyberg and her work are gifts to nursing leaders, health care systems, and ultimately to the public itself. Creating a caring path for administering a more caring and compassionate system, while still being accountable for organizational management, costs, and economic forces, make this a book for its time.

These ideas set forth the pathway and patterns for what is yet to come: a transformed, truly integrated health care organizational model—an organization that is guided by leaders and followers as partners, informed and transformed by an ethic of the whole, grounded in human caring values, processes, and outcomes that go deeper, last longer, and work. This book works for all these reasons and more.

Preface

Nursing Administration, the Beginnings

To get a perspective to begin the study of nursing administration, it seems appropriate to ground ourselves in our history. Our problems and our strengths are rooted in what our predecessors did and were, and what we build can be more appropriate and effective if we understand nursing administration as an evolving role.

From the dawn of civilization, as M.P. Donahue (1985) wrote, evidence supports the premise that nurturance is essential to the preservation of life. The practice of nursing came from the idea of a mother nursing her child. The role gradually expanded to envelope care of the sick, aged, helpless, and handicapped, as well as the general promotion of good health. "Care eventually encompassed affection, concern, and solitude, as well as responsibility for individuals in need" (p. 11). As time passed, it became apparent that love and caring alone were not sufficient to nurture health or overcome disease, so two other ingredients—skill/experience and knowledge—were added to nursing's repertoire.

Starr's (1982) extensive review of the history of American medicine says little about nursing but reveals much about how medicine climbed to a high social and financial level. It is instructive to recognize how nursing failed where medicine succeeded in becoming a powerful force in society.

Starr points out that medical professional power ascended from two basic sources: legitimacy and dependency. In the early 1900s, medicine had no status in America; that was changed by controlling the schools of medicine. Fly-by-night schools of medicine were shut down, and control of medical schools was brought under the university systems. About the same time, it was recognized that schools of nursing also should fall under the universities; such a change was not supported by medicine, which was busy trying to stake out its own place in society. Power for physicians also was greatly augmented in 1906, when the Pure Food and Drug Act channeled all drugs through medical doctors. With the advent of hospitals in the early 1900s, doctors solidified their control of medical care. By augmenting demand and controlling supply, physicians gained greater professional authority. They became the gatekeepers of medical services.

By the 1920s, enough scientific knowledge had been discovered for people to seek health care on their own. Physicians organized to become— and remain—a powerful lobby in Washington. Nurses have tried to organize for the last thirty years, but with less success than doctors.

In the early 1900s, the general public wanted more medical care than the medical system could provide. That key fact set up the history of high demand for health care. At that time, 4 percent of the United States gross national product went to health care. By the mid-1950s, two thirds of our population had medical insurance, and the demand for health care continued to grow. Doctors continued as the gatekeepers, and banded together into specialties, which further enhanced their status. In Starr's view, specialization brought the need for technical assistants, so doctors used women (nurses) who would not challenge their authority. Physicians' success as a group has remained firm by:

1. controlling the number of doctors

2. controlling ancillary health workers (nurses, physical therapists, chiropractors, optometrists)

3. controlling access to hospital services

4. remaining aloof

5. heavy lobbying

6. demanding fee-for-service reimbursement

7. maintaining a collegial structure

Nurses, the faithful care-givers, did nothing to secure their place in health care, as they were trained (mostly by doctors) to be handmaidens to physicians. People with money were cared for at home (good work for nurses, if they could get it), and the disenfranchised in society made up the patient and nurse populations at hospitals. During the Civil War, Clara Barton and Dorothea Dix cleaned up nursing and it became respectable to be a nurse. During each war, nurses were in short supply, and after the wars, nursing seemed to progress.

Erickson (1980), writing about the early years of nursing administration, contended that the status of the nursing superintendent in the early years had much to do with the progression of nursing. The first superintendents of nursing had a great deal of power and literally made the hospitals run smoothly. Unfortunately, these early nursing leaders did little planning about nursing's future; they ignored the proposal to put schools of nursing in universities. Now, a century later, the issue of nursing education remains unresolved.

Erickson noted that the superintendents of nursing ran the day-to-day affairs of the hospital, often being in contact with the hospital board of directors. Along with this responsibility, the superintendents were responsible for training all the student nurses. As medicine and nursing became more complex, the superintendents found themselves spread too thin. World War II brought about dramatic changes in nursing. With the advent of antibiotics, surgery, and x-rays, nurses' work became much more complex. There were not enough nurses to care for all the ill and wounded, and an impression grew that nursing superintendents were not capable of coping with the growing complexity of the hospital.

By the 1950s, the reputation of nursing directors was so tarnished that even nurses did not support them. Enter the hospital administrator. It was thought that a businessman's touch was needed to run the increasingly frenetic hospital. And since that time, the reputation of the nursing administrator has bobbed up and down.

That historical point of view has relevance today. It reminds us that nursing leaders have been at the top, the bottom, and in between. It helps us understand that our actions have far-reaching consequences. Many nurse executives have reached the top again, having direct contact with boards of directors and serving as a part of the corporate leadership of multinational corporate companies. I applaud their achievements and their skills. But, as our sisters of the past remind us, it is hard to be all things to all people. We must seek to provide values, standards, and theory to underpin the important but evolving mission of nursing administration.

The histories of medicine and nursing are very important at this crucial juncture in history. In some ways, doctors are losing power and nurses are gaining it. In other ways, both are losing power as insurance companies take on the job of rationing health care. But we should never forget that the work of nursing and medicine will always be symbiotic. In the immediate future, it will take the voices of doctors and nurses together to maintain caring values and beat back the brutality of the bureaucracy and the frustration that will come as health care is reformed.

I do not know what the health care system will look like in just a few years. But I know it will include many challenges and changes. It is a time for nursing to be an assertive participant in creating this new health care model. We must be expert business people, but it is also our responsibility to keep caring in the system. When people read the history of nursing a generation from now, how will it read? I believe that it is a time for nurse leaders to take control of maintaining the caring our practice has always held dear. I hope that this book can be instrumental in giving nurse administrators the confidence, knowledge, and skills needed to shape caring health care systems for the future.

Jan J. Nyberg

References

Donahue, M.P. (1985). *Nursing: The Finest Art.* St. Louis: C.V. Mosby.

Erickson, E.H. (1980). The nursing service director. *The Journal of Nursing Administration* 10 (4): 6–13.

Starr, P.P. (1982). *The Social Transformation of American Medicine.* New York: Basic Books.

Acknowledgments

I want to acknowledge the profound effect that the work and person of Dr. Jean Watson has had on me and my writing of this book. I met Dr. Watson in the late 1980s when I was a nurse executive and she was dean of the University of Colorado School of Nursing. I learned about caring from studying her written works, and I learned how to live caring by watching her do the same. I am honored to be a faculty associate in her Center for Human Caring. In the center, I met Karen Holland, who has been wonderful to me and encouraging about my ideas of applying the caring theory to nursing administration.

I also want to acknowledge the inspiration I have received from Dr. Mary Farley. She taught me the fine art of teaching and encouraged me to integrate caring and management theory. Finally, I want to acknowledge the loving support of my family. I was computer illiterate until my husband, Bart, bought me a lap-top computer that allowed me to work on this book from my recliner chair. My daughter, Cami, has graciously tolerated my irritability when I was stuck in my writing and when I was writing so furiously that I ignored the world. My son, Gregg, is my best cheerleader: he insisted I see this project through.

So, the book is a product of many people and many influences. I only hope it will have an impact on nursing in this crucial time when nursing is facing its greatest challenges.

CHAPTER ONE

Introduction

Being a nurse administrator is a challenging, tough, exciting, meaningful, frightening, fun, difficult, rewarding, demanding job. It has its ups and downs, but it is never dull! This book is intended for the nurse administrator who needs a time of reflection, and it is intended for nurses who wish to become administrators. It will not be a text for learning the basic skills of management (such as how to interview or discipline or do performance evaluations), and it will not be a rehash of old nursing or management theory. Rather, this book will explore some of the dilemmas and ethics of administration, and it will review some of the newer management theories and how they may impact the practicing administrator.

Since this book is about caring, part of the goal is that the book be caring. This requires a relationship of sorts between the writer and the reader. Therefore, I will write in the first person. As I share myself in these pages, I hope you will feel the passion I have for caring and for nursing administration, and I hope my experiences and thinking will be meaningful for you. The goal of the book is to use caring theory to develop some theoretical yet pragmatic ways of thinking about nursing administration that can be an anchor in the difficult days of everyday administration.

My qualifications for writing this book include:

1. Twelve years as a staff nurse.
2. Two years as a middle manager.
3. Five years as an associate director of nursing.
4. Five years as a chief nurse executive.
5. Six years as an assistant professor teaching nursing administration.
6. Several years as a consultant for nursing administration.
7. A master's degree in nursing administration.
8. A Ph.D. in nursing complex systems and organizations.
9. A deep, abiding love of the work of nursing administration and great respect for the people in that role.

The years I spent as a nurse administrator were my happiest professionally. I started work as an associate director of nursing right after finishing my master's degree in nursing administration. The hospital was a good one, but nursing was behind the times, so it became a workshop for my boss and me. The nursing organization was ripe for change in nursing, and we took advantage of that. Our first projects were setting up a quality assurance program, creating a patient classification system, and piloting primary nursing. Not bad for a year and a half's goals!

Since I had returned to school for my bachelor's degree at thirty years of age, I took my learning very seriously. And after obtaining my master's degree, I took my academic learning to work with me. I used conceptual models in most of my projects; it became a standing joke that I nearly wore out the photocopy machine distributing articles to the nurse managers on a regular basis. While some of our projects were more successful than others, the most important thing we did was to trigger excitement about nursing. When we were named a Magnet Hospital (a national study that identified the forty-one hospitals most highly regarded for their nursing services) in 1982, we were very proud.

At the interviews for the Magnet Hospital study, I compared ideas with other successful nurse administrators. We found that there were certain similarities in the ways we managed. First, we all placed great emphasis on the staff. We encouraged them, recognized the importance of their work, and rewarded them whenever we could. The feedback from the staff nurses who were interviewed for the study (apart from the nurse administrators) was that they felt valued. The other characteristic most noted by the staff nurses was that they saw their nurse administrators as visible and accessible. We all did things like making patient rounds, spending a day with a staff nurse, and developing staff nurse committees that had real input into decision making in nursing.

When I left administration and began teaching, I took those lessons with me. When I teach, I talk about the importance of contact with staff nurses and the use of conceptual models. As I journeyed through my Ph.D. program and began teaching and consulting, I still tried hard to teach the theories, but to ground them in reality as well. That will be the goal for this book. It will be heavily referenced because I find a great deal of help from old and new books and articles. It will also stay close to reality as I intersperse my experiences throughout the book.

Watson (1979, 1985) wrote two books about "caring" that have greatly affected my thinking on nursing. In her first book, she laid the groundwork of the caring theory. In her second book, Watson defined caring as a theory because "it helps me to see more broadly (clearly), and it may be useful in solving some conceptual and empirical problems in nursing and in human sciences generally." She defined a theory as "an imaginative grouping of knowledge, ideas, and experience that are represented symbolically and seek to illuminate a given phenomenon" (1985, p. 1). Watson's theory of caring is the grounding of this book. Communicating the concept of caring is my aim and purpose. For many years, I have been saying, "Caring is wonderful in the patient-nurse relationship, but how can that caring be sustained if the leaders do not also make caring a priority?" This book is written in a sincere attempt to encourage nurse administrators to make caring their goal in their work and in their lives.

As a discipline, nursing has been conservative about calling things "theory." Conversely, in business management there are lots of "theorists." In nursing we have recognized only about a dozen theorists in the last twenty years. In management, anyone who writes two or three articles is a theorist. In nursing administration, we have not really identified theorists. I believe we need to address some things more theoretically.

I do not claim to be nursing's great new theorist. Nonetheless, I hope to explore several concepts with the goal of creating at least a theoretical framework that addresses the important work of nursing administration. The basic concepts that will be explored in this book are: 1. Caring Theory; 2. Organization Theory; 3. Leadership Styles; 4. The Health Care

System; 5. Economic Theory; 6. Values and Ethics; 7. Research; and 8. Organizational Effectiveness. The conceptual assumptions for the book include:

1. *Person* is an integrated human being who has biological, psychological, sociological, and spiritual components, and these components interact to make a unique, valuable, and whole person. The person lives and is interconnected with the environment and universe.

2. *Health and illness* are described in terms of a dynamic, fluctuating continuum of well-being. Health and illness have physical, psychological, and spiritual facets. One can be physically well and yet not be healthy, and one can be physically ill and yet be healthy. Health is experienced as a harmony of mind/body/spirit and relationships. The potential for growth toward health depends on many factors in the person's life.

3. *Nursing* is a relationship between patient and nurse in which the nurse utilizes knowledge and skills to provide care and commits to caring for the patient as a holistic human being. Nursing is a valuable societal service and is based on the concept of human caring. Nursing has the ability to affect how patients experience their life-state.

4. *Environment* is a broad term signifying the physical, social, and behavioral attributes that interact to define reality for each unique person. Environment is an important contributor to health or illness. We have an immediate environment in our physical surroundings and a broader environment that includes social and political factors. Relationships should be considered as part of our environment because the human-environment unity is affected by the subjective world of the experiencing person.

5. *Nursing administration* is a specialty in nursing that has its own body of knowledge and practice roles. The nurse administrator uses knowledge of caring, nursing, and management to perform his/her job.

6. *Nursing administrative practice* is creating, monitoring, and evaluating systems for the practice of nursing. Its practice is influenced by underlying philosophies, values, theories, and knowledge. Those values are learned throughout life, but they can be influenced by new learning and experience.

7. *Nurse administrators* can make a difference in how nurses practice by developing systems and work environments that encourage autonomy and creativity and caring nursing practice. Quality nursing practice systems can lead to improved patient, family, and community health.

As my thoughts about administration have evolved, I have recognized that certain parts of the literature can give us a great deal of information that can be useful in our jobs. For example, out of my vigorous studies of nursing and organizational theory, I have chosen for this book the material that is most relevant to nursing administration now. So, I am not spending a great deal of time with other organizational theories such as classical, contingency management, ecology or natural selection, or environmental theories. This is not to say that these are unimportant, they just are not where I want to put my emphasis. First I will focus on the more contemporary organizational theorists that describe organizations of today and tomorrow, and I will also describe how some leadership styles are compatible with caring. Next I will write about bureaucracy and the health care system because I believe it still has a very great impact on our jobs.

Another important concept is economics. I will write about the budget process, the how-to-do economics, but I will give more attention to what impact economics has had and will have into the future. When considering the concepts of values and ethics, I will focus on how different value systems affect the practice of nursing administration. I will spend some time on research, and on organizational effectiveness/quality control. There will be discussion of the organization of nursing work and a definition the practice of *caring* nursing administration. We will think about the real mission of health care and determine how to optimize that mission. In order to bring some clarity to the overall book, I have constructed a model (Model 1.1) which shows the pieces of the puzzle and how they fit together.

At the top of the model is caring—my primary theme for the book. The overall question is this: "How can caring permeate our thinking about organizations, and how can it change the way we practice nursing administration?" In the model, the fluttering lines from the caring box visualize how the caring theory extends its influence on all other parts of the model. Caring is the theory—the anchor for evaluating literature and practice in nursing administration.

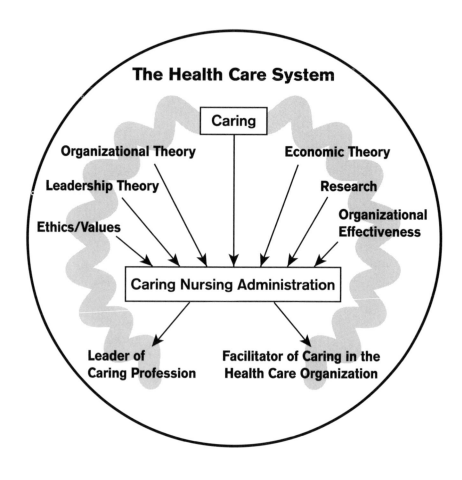

MODEL 1.1

The next six content areas on the model are the concepts that I believe are most importance in building a caring theory for nursing administration. They lead us to the caring solutions.

At the bottom of the model is the practice of nursing administration. It branches into two major functions: 1. leader of caring profession, and 2. facilitator of caring in the health care organization. The implications of these roles will be explored later.

Paradigms

Before we consider the main content areas, it is important to discuss the concept of paradigms. Throughout this book, you will find references to paradigms. Some years ago, Capra (1983) used the word to describe certain belief systems that affect the way we view life, death, and even the world around us. For example, he described a mechanistic paradigm (world view) where everything—including the human body—can be understood by viewing life as a machine that can be dismantled and studied in parts. This paradigm is problematic because it loses sight of the patient as a human being with thoughts and feelings—more than the sum of its parts. The biomedical model fits the mechanistic paradigm: it views the body as a machine that can be analyzed in terms of its parts. It therefore treats illnesses as diseases in the physical system that can be treated by killing them with drugs or cutting them out by surgery. Traditionally, organizations are also studied as mechanistic systems. For example, work engineering studies tasks and breaks them down into each movement used to complete the task. Managers were taught to study each organizational system as an independent unit, and there was little emphasis on the human part of the organization.

An alternative paradigm is the organistic view. This belief system sees the world as a growing, changing, interdependent interaction between multiple components that make up a whole that is different from the sum of its parts. It recognizes individuals as flexible, plastic living systems that are part of a larger system. The behavior of the individual parts, in fact, can be so unique and irregular that it bears no relevance to the order of the whole system. In the organistic paradigm, the ability to adapt to a changing environment is an essential characteristic.

The interpretation of health care is greatly affected by the paradigm being used. In the mechanistic paradigm there is a split between mind and body, and it loses sight of the patient as a whole human being. However, the majority of illnesses cannot be understood in terms of reductionist concepts of well-defined disease entities and single causes. The organistic or system paradigm has a new vision of reality that is based on awareness of the essential interrelatedness and interdependence of all phenomena—physical, biological, psychological, social, and cultural. Thus, illness is seen as a disruption of the organistic flow and the nature of the whole—which is always different from the mere sum of its parts.

The human organism is seen as a living system whose components are interconnected. Health, then, is an experience of well-being resulting from a dynamic balance involving the physical and psychological aspects of the organism, as well as its interactions with its natural and social environments. Organizations can also be viewed as living, interacting entities that have qualities that are more than the sum of their parts.

In business, there is also a movement to study and understand organizations in an organistic way. Attention is being given to values and ethics in management, and there is a lot written about how to work with employees as relating beings.

Kuhn (1970) studied paradigms and found that a prevailing paradigm will be the way people view reality until problems in understanding develop. As more and more problems arise that cannot be explained by the paradigm, there is pressure to formulate a new paradigm that explains the problems.

Currently, in health care, a paradigm shift is occurring. Just treating physical illnesses can leave the patient still unhealthy, if health is defined as a sense of wholeness and well-being. We are beginning to understand, for example, that extreme stress can be related to physical illness. Nurses have always viewed patients as holistic beings who need treatment as human beings, not just as illnesses. Capra acknowledges that a kind of primary care is being forcefully advocated today by nurses who are at the forefront of the holistic health movement.

This is important to understand because the caring part of nursing is aligned with the newer organistic paradigm. We still exist with one leg planted in a mechanized view of medicine and business, but the other leg is stepping forward into the newer holism. Capra wrote that nurses are well-prepared to meet the requirements of primary care: that we will play an important role in keeping the personal contact with the patient, integrating the special treatments into a meaningful whole. I believe nurse administrators can have a major effect on viewing the organization as a living system. Organizations are dependent on environmental variables, and they function as human organisms, not as machines.

This transition is very difficult for some nurses who have been heavily involved in science, medical care, and business principles. Yet many other nurses are finding in the new paradigm a place of belonging—a place where they can respond to patients as whole human beings who need

A Caring Approach in Nursing Administration

treatment of their person, not just their disease. Human caring is clearly a part of the new organistic paradigm. Organizational theory has moved along into a framework that is compatible with the caring theory.

When the word "paradigm" was first used, it referred to a whole belief system, a way to view the world. Since that time, "paradigm" has become a less intensive term. It is used commonly used to describe differences of opinions or streams of thought. "Paradigm," we will find, has found its way into many subject matters that will be covered in this book. And so we begin the journey of understanding caring theory in nursing administration. I hope it is a meaningful trip for us all.

References

Capra, F. (1983). *The Turning Point: Society and the Rising Culture*. New York: Bantam Books.

Kuhn, T. (1970). *The Structure of Scientific Revolutions*. Chicago: University of Chicago Press.

Watson, J. (1985). *Human Science and Human Care*. Norwalk, CT: Appleton-Century-Crofts.

————. (1979). *Nursing: The Philosophy and Science of Caring*. Boulder, CO: Colorado Associated University Press.

CHAPTER TWO

Caring and the Nursing Administrator

One of the foundational concepts for this book is that of caring. Caring is referred to throughout our society—it helps advertise hamburger, weight-loss systems, flowers, and clothing. Lots of commercials say "we care," but just what does that mean? We talk about caring about people—our moms, our children, our spouses, and our friends. There has been a lot written on caring. As we review the literature, we will focus on a couple of non-nurse writers and then several nurse authors.

Noddings (1984) wrote about caring as a feminine ethic. She was an educator, so she focused on the teacher-student relationship. She viewed caring as an extension of "natural caring" like a mother cares for a child. She wrote that it is our duty to maintain a preparedness to care that, for her, focuses on the welfare, protection, or enhancement of the one cared for. To care is to feel with another and involves the commitment of energy to the other. Caring is receiving the other unto oneself and sensing with and understanding the other. Noddings believes that caring and nurturing are traits more highly developed in women, who define their very reality in terms of caring relationships. She believes that this caring is a form of ethics, and that it is important—if not essential—to the future of our society.

Mayeroff (1971) was a philosopher who wrote a short book on caring. He says that "to care for another person, in the most significant sense is to help him grow and actualize himself" (p. 1). Mayeroff emphasizes that caring is primarily related to growth—of both people, but particularly for the one cared for. He defines caring ingredients as: knowing, alternating rhythms, patience, honesty, trust, humility, hope, and courage. Mayeroff wrote that, in the context of caring, one finds an ordering of life that results in stability and meaning. Thus, caring becomes a purpose and philosophy that determines how one lives and what consists of life's reward.

Nurses who have written about caring include Watson (1979, 1985), Leininger (1986), Ray (1989), Gaut (1983), Larson (1984), Valentine (1989), Swanson (1993), and others. Each has their own emphasis. For example, Gaut wrote that caring requires action. One is caring only if one takes action to help the one cared for. Leininger (1986) wrote extensively about caring as "the essence of nursing," and an essential human need for the full development, health maintenance, and survival of human beings in all world cultures. Ray (1981) developed a philosophical analysis within nursing. She, too, views caring as the central philosophical belief of nursing. Her analysis located the scope of caring by use of historical and contemporary sources of information and philosophies about human encounters. She also wrote about caring in intensive care units. She found that nurses in the intensive care units were very caring about their patients in spite of (and sometimes in consort with) all the machinery involved.

Watson has written two books about caring in nursing. In her first book (1979), she focuses on the foundations of caring and defined ten "carative" factors:

1. The formation of a humanistic-altruistic system of values.
2. The installation of faith-hope.
3. The cultivation of sensitivity to one's self and to others.
4. The development of a helping-trusting relationship.
5. The promotion and acceptance of the expression of positive and negative feelings.
6. The systematic use of the scientific problem-solving method for decision making.
7. The promotion of interpersonal teaching-learning.

8. The provision for a supportive, protective, and (or) corrective mental, physical, sociocultural, and spiritual environment.
9. Assistance with the gratification of human needs.
10. The allowance for existential-phenomenological forces.

(Watson 1979, p. 9–10)

In later editions, Watson changed number six ("the systematic use of the scientific problem-solving method for decision making") to "creative problem solving," which reflects the newer organistic paradigm for nursing. She also changed number ten ("the allowance for existential-phenomenologic forces") to "existential-phenomenological spiritual forces." I believe that including the word "spiritual" makes sense to more people than just, existential-phenomenological forces.

In Watson's (1985) second book, she describes the transpersonal caring experience. This is a special relationship in which the nurse enters into the lived experience of another person, and that person enters into the nurse's experience. Transpersonal caring relationship is a union with another, and contains a high regard for the whole person and their being in the world. In a nursing transpersonal experience, the involvement of the nurse is directed toward the other's self. The nurse affirms the subjective significance of the other person, assesses and realizes the other's condition of being-in-the-world, and feels a union with the other, causing the other to be able to have a release of some disharmony of the mind, body, and soul. This allows the person to direct pent-up energy to his or her own healing process.

In her second book, Watson also focuses more on what caring means to nursing and society. She writes of the "human-to-human care process of nursing" (p. viii). Part of Watson's desire is stated as, "I want nursing to move beyond objectivism, verification, rigid operations, and concern itself more with meaning, relationships, context, and patterns" (p. 2). So Watson's theory is phenomenological and metaphysical. She does not discount "hard science," but she clearly wants her own work to be more intuitive, culturally defined, and relational. Watson calls for a new lens for nursing that would help us appreciate some of its beauty, art, and humanity as well as its science. She calls her work "human science," which attempts to study the person as a whole.

Watson (1990) wrote that nursing is in a dramatic transition and is already in the process of being redesigned. We are seeking to bring about a

new consciousness of what it means to be a nurse—to be caring—
working toward a new social order where nursing and caring can exist or
at least coexist along with the technology and cure oriented order of
today. Nursing is accepting some new options about the notion of caring
and how it relates to health and healing. Watson says that "while caring
and traditional treatment can and perhaps must be present when curing is
called for, certainly caring must be present when curing has failed, and
death with dignity is the last result" (1990). The nurse carries a caring
consciousness that will help point the way toward certain human caring
actions that will direct the nurse's behavior in specific occasions.

Watson also wrote that the scholarly activities of nursing should not
be divorced from its clinical practice. The challenge of this book will be to
identify applicable theory and make it more pragmatic or real.

Watson says that nursing, as a human science, is threatened and frag-
ile. At this time in history, many nurses—and perhaps especially nursing
administrators—are in a precarious position. There are many new legislative initiatives that will be unsettled for some years to come. Indeed we
have never recovered from the 1983 government program called diagnosis-related groupings (DRG) system. But, as I recall, Starr (1982) said that
the first economic crisis in health care took place in 1914, and that helps
me to know that we cannot be paralyzed by fear. We must be aggressively
participating in the constant health care financial crisis.

In the next few years, caring will either be recognized as a valid business strategy, or it will be viewed as "fluff" we can no longer afford. Watson wrote that "Caring is the moral ideal of nursing whereby the end is
protection, enhancement, and preservation of human dignity" (1985,
p. 29). For me, caring is not "fluff." It is an undeniable and unquenching
need of the human soul, and therefore nursing can never give up on it.
Caring is standing shoulder to shoulder with those in need (in nursing,
mostly health needs) and being part of improving their human status.
And for the nurse administrator, it is being caring oneself and working to
make health care more caring as a system that really matters.

Watson believes that a recognition and acknowledgment of the value
of human care in nursing comes before and presupposes actual caring. We
should not assume that nurses are practicing human care when they practice nursing:

The ideal and value of caring is not just a "thing" out there, but is a starting point, a stance, an attitude which has to become a will, an intention, a commitment and a conscious judgment that manifests itself in concrete acts. . . . Nursing is the profession that has an ethical and social responsibility to both individuals and society to be the caretaker of care and the vanguard of society's human care needs now and in the future.

(1985, p. 32)

In Watson's (1994) later writings, she said that the human caring process in nursing is a special, delicate gift to be cherished. She believes that fundamental clinical, technological competencies and knowledge are a necessity to caring. This is an important point, since some nurses believe that "there is more to nursing than caring," referring to nursing skills. To Watson, skills are a requisite to caring, not separate from it. Benner and Wrubel (1989) agree that caring is always understood in a context. When the situation calls for technical proficiency, then technical proficiency is experienced as caring. When the patient situation does not call for technical actions, expressive actions such as recognizing the patient's uniqueness are identified as caring.

Bevis and Watson (1989) call for changes in education whereby caring would be emphasized. They advocate demonstration projects of expert human caring, healing, and health. They would like to see a mix of nurses with different levels of participation who would be initiated to test out and demonstrate quality, efficiency, and cost effectiveness. These models should be tested in hospitals and other agencies across the country.

Eriksson (1989) studied student nurses when they began their studies and at the end of their studies. While in school, they were introduced to caring theory. She found that nurses can act according to external technical facts or to deep internal interests of caring. She wrote that there have been times, especially during the dominant medical and multidisciplinary periods, when the attributes of caring disappeared. The mission of education is to help students to understand caring attributes and form an opinion about them and then develop caring in their practice. The students in this study all stated that they would have liked to develop their practice toward more concentration on caring and the patient as a human being. The greatest differences at the end of the study were

A Caring Approach in Nursing Administration

increased ability to communicate caring capability and to evaluate what really good caring was.

Watson (1994) views the process of caring as illuminating the mystery of humanity and the possibility of a higher power, order, or energy in the universe. This, in turn, can potentiate healing and health and facilitate self-knowledge, self-reverence, self-control, self-care, and the possibility of even self-healing. This extends caring past just a day-to-day practice. Watson views caring as "the moral ideal of nursing. Human caring consists of transpersonal, intersubjective attempts 1. to protect, enhance, and preserve humanity by helping a person find meaning in illness, suffering, pain, and existence; 2. to help another gain self-knowledge, self-control, and self-healing" (p. 220).

Caring is the central issue for Benner and Wrubel (1989) in *The Primacy of Caring*. They describe caring as a way of being in the world. They believe that the devaluation of nursing care comes from our highly technical society that values autonomy, individualism, and competitiveness. Caring is that "soft" part of our culture where people exchange pieces of their souls with one another. "The goal is to achieve a nursing science that examines the lived experience of human illness and the relationships among health, illness, and disease" (p. xvi). Benner and Wrubel describe caring as essential in a world where some things matter and others do not. Caring makes the nurse notice when interventions help and when signs of improvement or deterioration take place. "Caring is primary because it sets up the possibility of giving and receiving help" (p. 4). Non-caring is not to be present with the patient, but rather being there "only to get the job done" (p. 5). These authors feel strongly that caring can alter the state of health, illness, and disease. Caring is understanding the meaning of the illness for that person: "Such understanding can overcome the sense of alienation, loss of self-understanding, and loss of social integration that accompany illness" (p. 9). "The nurse has to, in some sense, personally come to terms with the reality of the illness and is able to convey acceptance and understanding to the patient" (p. 112). Benner and Wrubel wrote that getting to know the patient's story is often just a beginning— knowing what the illness interrupted and understanding the symptoms helps see the patient in context. They emphasize that "more than any other helping professionals, nurses attend to the relationship between illness and disease . . . This relationship can never be a simple one of mind over matter or of body over mind because the mind and the body are not dual realities" (p. 21). Not only do nurses want to be cared for; it is of utmost importance for them to feel that their work is set up to allow them to express care to their patients. As Benner and Wrubel say:

> We maintain that if nurses were liberated to give the care that they want to give and were able to use their knowledge in a fully efficacious way, while being adequately rewarded, the stresses inherent in nursing would be reduced to the manageable level imposed by the legitimate demands inherent in caring. The stress of nursing becomes intolerant when the demands of the situation prevent the nurse from performing with a maximum level of skill and compassion.
>
> (Benner and Wrubel 1986, p. 369)

Benner and Wrubel identify three components involved in caring: 1. creating a climate for establishing a commitment to healing, 2. presencing— offering one's full and conscious attentiveness to every encounter, and 3. guiding patients through emotional and developmental changes.

Swanson (1993) wrote about "nursing as informed caring for the well-being of others." She maintains that people are unique beings who are in the midst of becoming and whose wholeness is made manifest in thoughts, feelings, and behaviors (p. 352). She sees that nursing knowledge is sometimes hidden in caring acts, and the acts are often hidden, undervalued, and underrewarded. She says that it takes a person "schooled in nursing appreciation" to fully see the beauty in expert nursing practice. She believes that the practice of nurses is grounded in nursing knowledge, related to the humanities as well as to personal insight and experiential understanding. Swanson defines five caring practices:

1. Maintaining belief—an orientation to caring requires a fundamental belief in a person's capacity to make it through events and transitions and face a future with meaning.

2. Knowing—an anchor that moors the beliefs of nurses to the lived realities of those being cared for.

3. Being with—conveys to clients that they matter to the nurse. To be with another is to give time, authentic presence, attentive listening, and reflective responses.

4. Doing for—comforting the other, anticipating their needs, performing competently and skillfully, protecting the other, and preserving the dignity of the one being cared for.

5. Enabling—includes coaching, informing, explaining to the other, supporting the other, and enabling others to practice self-care.

Thus, for Swanson, caring is "grounded in maintenance of a basic belief in persons, anchored by knowing the other's reality conveyed through being with, and enacted through doing for and enabling" (p. 357).

Sherwood (1997) wrote that a health care revolution is sweeping the United States which is threatening the core values of caring. She challenges nurses to have the courage to maintain caring as the foundation of nursing. She says that the human element—experiencing connectedness with patients and nurses—is the satisfier in nursing's work, and that failure to experience connectedness results in isolation and dissatisfaction in one's life.

Caring is equally important to patients. Williams (1997) did a study about the relationships of patients' perceptions of satisfaction with nursing care. She found a significant positive relationship between patients' perceptions of nursing caring and their satisfaction with nursing care.

Sherwood describes the guiding principles of caring:

1. Caring as Individuality: having awareness of another's unique person. It is communicated through actions such as eye contact, body language, and tone of voice. These actions take no additional time yet make a difference in patient well-being.

2. Caring as Presence: acknowledges a shared humanity—a connection with another that goes beyond tasks.

3. Caring as Knowing: "knowledgeable caring is the highest form of commitment in giving patient care" (p. 33). Knowledge entails knowing both the scientific and the caring needed to be a truly competent nurse.

4. Caring as Interacting: establishing human connectedness for therapeutic outcomes. It enhances growth, restores, reforms, and potentiates learning and healing.

Sherwood concludes that:

Nurses possess caring values at a universal level and are called upon to honor, preserve, protect, and be proud of them if the profession is to survive. Caring is acting out of positively intentional actions, having awareness of need with an intent to make a positive difference. It is expressed by taking a specific set of actions or interventions based on sound knowledge and judgment. This is carried out through connection, an interaction of mutuality, and interconnectedness between recipient and care giver (p. 36).

Boykin and Schoenhofer (1993) wrote that their basic premise is that all persons are caring, and caring is an essential feature and expression of being human. Like Sherwood, these authors believe that there is little in the health care environment to support caring at the present time. There are five major concepts of caring: 1. a human trait; 2. a moral imperative; 3. an effect; 4. an interpersonal interaction; and 5. an intervention. Boykin and Schoenhofer believe caring is a process in which persons grow in their ability to express caring. Caring can be expressed even during uncaring procedures, and non-caring can be expressed while doing caring acts. This is important because it confirms my experience of seeing people grow in their ability to express caring: caring is not only an innate ability. The ability to express caring varies in the moment and develops over time. This should be encouraging to nurse administrators who want caring to be actualized in their organizations. All relationships are opportunities for caring. The nurse administrator who uses caring in all his/her relationships will do much to promote caring throughout the organization. Teachers and consultants may also be used to teach and model caring to nurses at all levels.

Most nurses have an understanding of caring. The problem is often that the organizational environment does not value and reward caring experiences. Boykin and Schoenhofer write that "when one's 'nursing self' is a depersonalized, disembodied tool, nursing tends to lose its flavor and devoted commitment to nursing. This may lead to nurse burn-out" (p. 45). The nurse administrator would do well to focus on caring in an ongoing way.

To summarize the last few authors, caring has meaning in relationships with patients and with nurses. Some of the words used by scholars to describe caring make it seem esoteric and idealistic. But they have a way of making it seem very important, and it is. I agree with Sherwood and with Boykin and Schoenhofer that nurses possess caring values, but some are more tuned in to them and have a natural instinct to behave in a caring manner. I also believe that caring instincts can be enhanced and brought to the forefront of nurses' thinking and actions. I also believe that being caring is essential for nurse and patient satisfaction. The commitment to caring, however, must be supported by the nurses' work environment, and that is where nursing administrators come in. In addition to behaving in a caring manner, the administrator can set up systems to enhance caring throughout the organization.

While we are focusing on the word "caring," other terms can be used to describe the beliefs and behaviors of caring. The Pew-Fetzer Task Force (Tresolini 1994) issued a report that focused on "relationship-oriented care." The report says that there are palpable signs of a growing need to enhance the quality and care process from the perspective of both the patient and the practitioner. They feel that a primary focus on ways to enhance the relationships that are relative to health care should be addressed through education and practice. The foundation report says that the relationships are vitally important to both the care-giver and patient. They are a medium for the exchange of all forms in information, feelings, and concerns and an essential ingredient in the satisfaction of both parties. For patients, the relationship with their provider frequently is the most therapeutic aspect of the health care encounter. Thus, *relationship-centered care* should be a focus throughout health care. In order to develop such relationships, the practitioner needs technical knowledge and skills; the ability to attend to patient's dignity, integrity, and uniqueness; and the ability to compassionately respond to patients' distress and pain. Although Pew-Fetzer uses the term "relationship-oriented care," it is clearly a fine way to describe caring.

Montgomery (1993) wrote about the *practice* of caring, which is healing through communication. She emphasizes that caring is not an individual accomplishment in which the helper succeeds by achieving mastery over a client's problem; caring is expressed through meaningful participation in an experience with a client. Montgomery said that caring is contextual: it depends on the intensity of the circumstances, team participation, and patient participation. Examples of intense circumstances are the emergency rooms, recovery rooms, and operating rooms where the caring is instantaneous bonding and a heightened power of communication. In less intense contexts, the caring can be achieved in a slower, more considered manner.

Montgomery believes that caring is more likely to occur within teams that foster a web of supportive connections. She writes that "there's something about loving the nurses you work with that makes it easier to love patients" (p. 80). Caring is a patient-centered activity where the caregiver connects with the patient's center or inner spirit. Some nurses believe that they must keep an objective distance from patients so that they don't get overinvolved. Montgomery addressed this fear of getting "sucked out" or "losing it." She said that expert care-givers do not have to keep their distance from patients. They integrate their feelings with their own knowledge, experience, and support systems to achieve a therapeutic caring relationship. When the relationship is right, there is a flow, harmony, and easiness to caring, and the caring occurs from within a contextual web of connection. Caring can be an energizing peak experience that creates meaning and reinforces commitment, self-esteem, and feelings of personal empowerment for the patient and the nurse.

A few other authors address the need for technical skills in relation to caring. Montgomery writes that "not only does caring require the technical abilities and competencies of one's chosen field, but it also requires the courage to let one's heart enter into the experiences of great emotional risk, the strength to endure the pain, and the wisdom to be able to find meaning in the experience. Caring is an integral part of the process of healing" (p. 127). Montgomery emphasizes that it is essential for care delivery systems to allow for consistent personal involvement with patients and time to prioritize workloads based on caring rather than task completion: "If this is not done, increasing numbers of health care professionals will withdraw emotionally or leave the profession altogether because they find it impossible to care in the present system" (p. 133).

From the literature, we begin to get a picture of caring from the perspective of the authors. Caring is clearly something nurse-scholars have been considering for a long time. While all of the descriptions of caring have much in common, each author's description is different—kind of like several painters trying to paint the same subject. This is the beauty and uniqueness of caring—it's something we can all understand, but we only really understand it from our own frame of reference. It is, I think, the very *art* of nursing.

Sometimes I wish we could find a word other than "caring" because it is overused. I don't believe nursing has an exclusive corner on caring. I have known doctors, physical therapists, and other health care providers that know a lot about caring. One of the differences in caring in nursing is that it is the nurse who sees a patient at his/her most vulnerable times. We do things to and with patients that no one even likes to think about doing for themselves. Another difference is that we are with patients in a longer time frame than others. We are there twenty-four hours a day, seven days a week, and patients quickly learn that it makes little sense to hold anything back from their nurse. Lastly, there is a therapeutic part of our caring that is different than the baker, florist, or hamburger joint. A commercial business depends on making consumers happy, and nurses cannot always do that. Sometimes we have do things that hurt, and sometimes we have to tell people things they really do not want to hear. But that therapeutic part of caring distinguishes the care a nurse gives.

Little has been written about the association of nursing skills to nursing caring. As we have seen, most theorists just say that you can't be caring without being skilled—skills are a prerequisite for caring. I don't see things quite so simply. Being a nursing administrator for ten years gave me a long view of the development of nurses. Basically, I agree with Benner's *From Novice to Expert* (1984), which says that novice nurses focus their attention on the task before them. Sometimes I have seen young nurses do procedures without ever looking at the patient. They were just too focused on the skill to be able to relate to the patient at the same time. Then, I would see these nurses blossom into Benner's "advanced nurses" who could walk into a room and sense the whole of the situation. But there were many nurses stuck in the middle. They provide the bulk of the nursing care. And, unfortunately, they did not always advance in technical skills and caring skills at the same time. I always wondered what to do with a nurse who was very skilled and weak in caring or the other way around. There was one nurse who particularly perplexed me. Other nurses did not like to work with her because she was technically weak (not incompetent, just weak), and yet I got more lovely letters from her patients talking about what a wonderful, caring nurse she was. Our response was to work on her skills and praise her for caring. I am not so sure we gave equal concern, though, to the nurses who were technical whizzes and not very caring. We put them in ICU! To be committed to having a caring organization, there must be emphasis on growing as a caring nurse, not just a technical one.

As I read about caring as helping patients cope, of trying to understand what illness means to a person, it struck me that these same principles apply to the practice of nurse manager or nurse administrator. Their job is to intervene in the stresses and difficult life experiences of their primary patients—the nurses! Even though the patient care part of health care seems diminished by the economic parts, the nurse administrator must not let go of the immediacy of caring throughout the organization, as illness can alter the way a nurse feels about his/her work. Caring is as applicable to caring for nurses as it is for caring for patients.

So, if nursing is responsible for caring in society, what is the role of the nurse administrator? It is awesome, of course. Miller (1987) says that it is a constant challenge for the nursing administrator to create a climate for caring. And you cannot do that by issuing an order or memo. The nursing staff needs to feel that the caring starts with the nurse executive. Watson (1985) describes a "transpersonal" caring experience where two people closely connect and commit to each other. I believe that the nurse administrator must seek her own transpersonal caring moments. These mostly likely will occur with those she directly supervises, but it need not be restricted to those people. One of the last transpersonal experiences I had as a nurse administrator was with a child who was having severe pain. I certainly was not an expert in pain in children, but I took fifteen to twenty minutes to connect with that little boy. I used no magic tricks, I just touched him and soothed him and talked and sang to him. When I left, his mother stopped me. She was in tears herself, but she knew I had a special moment with her son, and she could see him sleeping peacefully.

It is not easy for a nurse administrator to find time for such caring moments. It seems like there is never an extra twenty minutes—people are after you all the time. But administrators need meaning in their lives, too. It is not enough to go from meeting to meeting and task to task. Nurses in all types of jobs need the reward of caring and being cared for.

To this point, we have focused on care in one-on-one relationships— the dyads of patient and nurse or nurse-administrator to one staff person. But, as much as nursing administrators need to forever keep that kind of caring in mind, nursing administrators have to translate caring to the systems level. We can still have our caring moments, but we must also set the stage for a caring organization.

There is a growing interest in caring at the organizational level. It was a bold new stance when Schultz (1987) wrote about the need to reconceptualize the client to include more than one. She believes that it is appropriate to focus nursing care on interaction groups such as families, groups, organizations, and communities. She points out that, on occasion, the decision to deliver health care to an individual (like a heart transplant) will preclude addressing health care for the community (like child immunization clinics).

This article had a big impact on me. I feel like most nurses—that I have always cared for my patients! But after I met Jean Watson, I had to *really* think about what caring meant to me as a nurse. I read and read and went about my administration trying to care more for each individual I encountered. But Schultz gave me the impetus to think that maybe nurses who deal with groups instead of individuals can still practice caring. That thought opened up all kinds of opportunities. As I went to a head-nurse group, I was aware that I could care for the group as well as the individuals in the group. Since much of my work was with groups, I urgently tried to incorporate caring into my work with groups. It made an amazing difference. It made a happier environment and yet a more open one. As I tried to care for the group, I found myself more capable of hearing about problems as well as good things. I felt much less like I had to solve all their problems; because as I cared for the group, I saw more potential for them to solve their own problems. Some groups were harder than others, of course, but the major difference was in how I felt about my work. I could practice caring at every turn, and that made work much more rewarding.

Fortunately for me, I had recently enrolled in the Ph.D. program at the University of Colorado School of Nursing. Dr. Schultz was my teacher, and so was Dr. Marilyn Ray. Ray was deeply committed to caring, and she had a special interest in how an organization could implement caring. She wrote an important article entitled "Health Care Economics and Human Caring in Nursing; Why the Moral Conflict Must Be Resolved." That represented what my job was all about: the dilemma of caring and economics. I spent my days trying to mesh the two, and the pressure was enormous. Ray believes that:

Defining the essence of caring in terms of commodities to be bought and sold in the marketplace appears incongruous; but in society, there is often a need to address two things simultaneously that are seemingly incompatible or mutually exclusive. For society, nurses must be not only be loyal to caring as a moral ideal in health care, but can also be responsible to society by involvement in the search to formulate the means to preserve human caring in an increasingly economic health delivery system.

(Ray 1987, p. 36)

Ray suggested that cost-benefit and cost effectiveness should include caring in their equation. She felt that a synthesis of economics and caring provides a way out of the conflict by legitimizing the expansion of economic models to include caring as a legitimate economic resource.

Ray wrote an article about bureaucratic caring in 1989. In that article she interviewed people in all different departments and found that most every person felt their work to be related to caring. It was somewhat difficult to equate the financial director's idea of how his work contributed to caring, but many people from different departments felt the same. It helped me to understand that an organization can have infighting between departments and yet all be working for the same goal—*caring.*

With the influence of Drs. Watson, Ray, and Schultz, I was hooked on caring. The title of my dissertation became *Human Care and Economics: A Nursing Study.* I spent the next couple of years trying to find some understanding about the dilemma that had plagued my work as a nursing administrator. I have not come up with any revolutionary answers, but I have discovered factors that I believe can increase the caring portion of an organization. Certain management literature, economic systems, and ethical positions can combine to enhance caring. These are presented later in this book.

About the time I really began working on researching economics and caring, I reached a terrible personal dilemma that affected my future work in nursing. I had developed a physical disability that forced me to give up my job as a nursing administrator. I was crushed. Oh, I had my bad days, but basically I really loved my job. The idea of not being able to be a nursing administrator was a cruel disappointment.

But sometimes things work out for the best. For the first time, I had time to really reflect on what my job had been and what it had meant to me. I decided that I wanted to do a study that would have meaning to me and to other nurse administrators. I knew that caring would be the primary concept.

When you decide to make caring a central element in your life, you can read and read. But there comes a time when you have to say to yourself, "Just what does this caring mean to me—how do I apply it to my life?" It was natural for me to consider caring as an administrator, but it took me weeks to really be able to articulate caring as my very own concept—my own reality of caring. The result of that thinking is in the following chapter.

References

Benner, P. (1984). *From Novice to Expert*. Menlo Park, CA: Addison-Wesley Publishing Co.

Benner, P., and J. Wrubel, (1989). *The Primacy of Caring*. Menlo Park, CA: Addison-Wesley Publishing Co.

Bevis, E., and J. Watson, (1989). A new paradigm of curriculum development. *Toward a Caring Curriculum: New Pedagogies for Nursing Education*. National League for Nursing, New York.

Boykin, A. and S. Schoenhofer, (1993). *Nursing as Caring: A Model for Transforming Practice*. New York: National League for Nursing Press.

Eriksson K. (1989). Caring paradigms: a study of the origins and the development of caring paradigms among nursing students. *Scandinavian Journal of Caring Science* 3 (4): 169–175.

Gaut, D. (1983). A theoretic description of caring as action. In Leininger, M. *Care: The Essence of Nursing and Health*. Detroit: Wayne State University Press. pp. 27–44.

Larson, P. (1984). Important nurse caring behaviors perceived by patients with cancer. *Oncology Nursing Forum* 11 (6): 46–50.

Leininger, M., ed. (1986). *Care: The Essence of Nursing and Health*. Detroit, MI: Wayne State University Press.

Mayeroff, M. (1971). *On Caring*. New York: Barnes and Noble Books.

Miller, K. (1987). The human care perspective in nursing administration. *The Journal of Nursing Administration* 17 (2): 10–12.

Montgomery, C. L. (1993). *Healing Through Communication: The Practice of Caring*. Newbury Port, CA: Sage Publications.

Noddings, N. (1984). *Caring: A Feminine Approach to Ethics and Moral Education*. Berkeley: University of California Press.

Ray, M. (1987). Health care economics and human care in nursing: Why the moral conflict must be resolved. *Family and Community Health*. 10 (1): 35–43.

———. (1982). A philosophic analysis of caring within nursing. In Leininger, M. *Caring: An Essential Human Need*. Detroit: Wayne State University Press, pp. 23–37.

———. (1989). The theory of bureaucratic caring for nursing practice in the organizational culture. *Nursing Administration Quarterly* 13 (2): 31–42.

Sherwood, G. (1997). Patterns of caring: the healing connection of interpersonal harmony. *Journal of Nursing Administration* 1 (1): 30–38.

Schultz, P. R. (1987). Clarifying the concept of "client" for health care policy formulation: ethical implications. *Family and Community Health* 10 (1): 73–82.

Starr, J. P. (1982). *The Social Transformation of American Medicine.* New York: Basic Books.

Swanson, K. M. (1993). Nursing as informed caring for the well-being of others. *Image* 25 (4): 352–357.

Tresolini, C. P., and the Pew-Fetzer Task Force. (1994). *Health Professions Education and Relationship-Centered Care.* San Francisco, CA: Pew Health Professions Commission.

Valentine, K. (1989). Caring is more than kindness. *Journal of Nursing Administration* 19 (11): 28–34.

Watson, J. (1985). *Human Science and Human Care.* Norwalk, CT: Appleton-Century-Crofts.

———. (1979). *Nursing: The Philosophy and Science of Caring.* Boulder, CO: Colorado Associated University Press.

———. (1990). Transpersonal caring: a transcendent view of person, health, and healing, *Nursing Theories in Practice.* New York: National League for Nursing.

———. (1989). Watson's philosophy and theory of human caring in nursing. *Conceptual Models for Nursing Practice,* 3rd edition. Ed., Riehl-Sisca. Norwalk, Conn.: Appleton and Lange.

———. (1994). Watson's philosophy and theory of human caring in nursing. *Conceptual Models for Nursing Practice,* 3rd edition. Norwalk, Conn.: Appleton and Lange.

Williams, S. A. (1997) The relationship of patients' perceptions of holistic nursing caring or satisfaction with nursing care. *Journal of Nursing Care Quality* 11 (5): 15–29.

CHAPTER THREE

The Element of Caring in Nursing Administration*

The term "caring" is commonly used among nurses to describe interactions between patients and other nurses. Can caring be defined, measured, or evaluated? Is it something that a person has naturally, or can it be developed? Is it a purely subjective experience, or can it have objective aspects as well? Surely everybody cares about others and about their work. Is caring more than the natural response to life? Can it be enhanced to make a difference in how nurses and administrators actually behave in daily life?

In this chapter we will explore the meaning as it has been defined in literature and as it can be experienced as a growing force in professional life. In particular, we will define caring as it can affect the emerging discipline of nursing administration.

In defining the term "caring" one can identify three different uses of the word. "Care" can be defined as a burden: "I have many cares in life"; as responsibility: "I will care for you"; and as a feeling toward another: "I

---

* Reprinted by permission from *Nursing Administration Quarterly* (1989); 13(3):9–16. © 1989 Aspen Publishers, Inc.

care deeply for you." In medicine, caring for a patient primarily involves taking responsibility to cure illness or solve health problems. Nurses are involved in the responsibility of the curing part of care, but they also practice caring in the emotional sense. On the whole, nurses care for and about patients. They provide technical and physical care, but they also establish relationships with their patients as individual human beings. In nursing, caring for patients is sometimes a burden, sometimes a responsibility, and sometimes a feeling toward the patient.

Noddings (1984) focuses on caring as a feminine approach to ethics and moral understanding. To practice the "caring ethic," one must maintain a preparedness to care, and in caring must focus on the welfare, protection, or enhancement of the cared-for. To care is to act, not by fixed rule, but by affection and regard. Caring involves feeling with the other, receiving the other unto oneself, sensing with and understanding the other. It also involves the commitment of energy to the service of the other. Caring is primarily relatedness and connectedness. And, as one cares for others and is cared for by them, caring for oneself is possible as well. Basic reality is defined in terms of caring relationships.

Mayeroff (1971) suggests that "to care for another person, in the most significant sense, is to help him grow and actualize himself" (p. 1). He describes caring as a process that emerges in time through mutual trust and a deepening of the relationship. He maintains that a person may care for many things, such as people, ideas, and communities. The common pattern is helping the other grow. Mayeroff's emphasis on helping other people to grow is not meant to be a dominating approach: "Instead of trying to dominate and possess the other, I want it to grow in its own right, or, as we sometimes say, 'to be itself,' and I feel the other's growth as bound up with my own sense of identity" (p. 6). In caring for someone or something, we must be able to sense that other's potential and need to grow; we must also believe in our ability to help the other to grow.

The earliest nurse theorist to recognize the concept of caring as it applies to nursing practice was Florence Nightingale, who stressed that nurses must be devoted to the very welfare of their patients. Other nurse theorists, such as Orem, Rogers, Peplau, and Henderson, also recognized the importance of the relational, interactive component of nursing. More recently, Watson (1979, 1985) has described caring as a "human science." This author broadens the perception of nursing beyond scientific principles toward a culturally defined process that emphasizes caring as central to its existence.

> Nursing science has to work at changing its lens to see anew and appreciate some of its beauty, art, and humanity as well as its science. Perhaps the issue for nursing is to acknowledge that it is not like the traditional sciences—it requires its own description, possesses its own phenomena, and needs its own method for clarification of its own concepts and their meanings, relationships and context.
>
> (Watson 1985, p. 8)

Leininger (1986) states that caring is the "essence of nursing" and advocates the study of caring in order to understand its meaning in nursing. Gaut (1983) performs a conceptual and theoretical analyses of caring and develops an action-based description of caring as an intentional human enterprise directed toward the goal of bringing about a positive change in the one who is cared for. Ray (1982) develops a philosophical analysis of caring within nursing, identifying the recurrent theme of growth or mutual self-actualization and the concepts of copresence and love. She also examines caring within the cultural context of the hospital, developing a classification system or taxonomy of caring as it applies to institutions.

From this variety of authors, the central characteristics of caring can be identified for the purpose of defining the term. Caring begins as an interest in someone, which expands through knowledge to a feeling and a commitment to assist the person to exist and grow. As one experiences the satisfactions of an individual caring relationship, caring becomes a part of one's philosophy and approach to life. Caring is a way of thinking and acting that determines more and more of an individual's behavior as they allow the intuitive, relating part of themselves to invade their awareness. As knowledge of caring is attained, each nurse applies this knowledge to his or her own area of practice. For the nurse administrator, caring is not confined to a patient-nurse relationship. It can be very useful in dealing with staff nurses and others in the context of the organization. The nurse administrator can exemplify caring and thus enrich the patient care environment by insisting on the development of an emphasis on caring behaviors throughout the nursing division.

How can such laudable goals be attained in management? Miller (1987) calls attention to the responsibility of the nurse administrator to set the tone for caring in health care facilities. But how does one go about becoming more caring? Perhaps this may be accomplished by developing the following attributes.

Attributes Conducive to Caring

For the nursing administrator, five attributes enable one consistently to exhibit caring behaviors: commitment, self-worth, ability to prioritize, openness, and ability to bring out potential. By understanding and developing these attributes, the nurse administrator can be the role model who exemplifies caring and encourages it to become an institutional norm.

Commitment

The first attribute, commitment, consists of three components: interest, knowledge, and commitment. Caring begins at the time a person first takes a special interest in someone. For an object of interest to evolve into an object of care, there must be a time of learning about the person that leads to a level of understanding and a desire to get involved more personally.

If the relationship evolves into one of understanding and trust, and if the potential care-giver feels willing and able to contribute to the growth of the other, a commitment may be made to care for the other. The last part of the phase of establishing the caring relationship is that the one who is cared for must be receptive and willing to be cared for.

The attribute of commitment is essential to the caring relationship. As Mayeroff points out, "caring is not always agreeable, it is sometimes frustrating and rarely easy" (p. 72). To care for someone, one must be committed to a continuing relationship. It can be very damaging for a person to be cared for briefly and then to be shut off from that caring. Subsequent trust in people may diminish, making it difficult for that person to accept care from others. Trust is a large part of the caring relationship, and it is established through the strength of the commitment of the caring person.

Self-Worth

The second attribute that promotes caring emphasizes the need for the nursing administrator to achieve feelings of self-worth, self-understanding,

A Caring Approach in Nursing Administration

and self-confidence. Many of the behaviors that detract from a caring manner are connected with anxiety about one's own security and place in life. If there is constant concern about meeting one's own needs for achievement, being accepted by others, or obtaining personal rewards, it is impossible to find energy and time to address the needs of others.

This area is one of great importance in organizational life. Many people become administrators because of an inner need to achieve a position of power and prestige that allows them to feel secure in their identity. A healthy need for achievement can be useful if it leads to feelings of personal success that can be shared by others. An inordinate drive to get to the top, however, can lead to disregard for others and the organization.

Rather than dealing privately with issues of self-worth, some administrators make the organization an arena in which to play out their personal issues. They may withhold rewards, be overly critical, or demand to be in charge of every situation. They often court the favor of people in the organization whom they believe can help them get ahead. It is not unusual for insecure administrators to have favorites on their staff who maintain the nurse administrator's power and control by never questioning or challenging him or her. Such administrators may stifle creativity and growth in others, because the others are perceived as competitive and threatening to the nurse administrator.

Another common issue regarding self-worth is that of placing importance on meeting one's personal and social needs. Unfortunately, the norm in many organizations is that the administrator works longer and harder than anyone else. Personal needs for outside friends, leisure activities and growth are subordinated to work priorities, and administrators become progressively dependent on organizational success to maintain their sense of identity and worth. Then, if something goes wrong in the organization, the administrator feels personally devastated, self-doubt is reinforced, and the cycle continues.

Attention to personal needs is very important for nursing administrators. One should never feel guilty about maintaining healthy activities outside of work. The reality is that only by doing so can one feel the inner stability that leads one to be caring as an administrator. The concept of caring requires that caring persons have developed a strong sense of self-worth, feel cared for in their own lives, and see themselves as having something to offer others through the caring process.

Prioritize

The third attribute that enables one to be caring is the ability to prioritize and order life's activities in a way that allows time and energy for the caring process. Mayeroff and Noddings talk about the need to limit caring relationships to a few significant others, in order to have time and energy to pay attention to one's own needs as well as the needs of others. This becomes a very difficult task for the nursing administrator, who has an abundance of people in the organization who need to be cared for. Some nursing administrators handle the situation by retreating into businesslike behavior and a bureaucratized method of managing by rules and policies. It is impossible to care for everyone, so they care for no one. While such a posture may help to insulate the administrator, the environment it produces is often rigid, impersonal, and inflexible. Nursing managers feel uncared for and pass this feeling on to staff nurses who pass it on to patients.

The nursing administrator can prioritize his or her job to encourage caring opportunities and reflect a caring approach. He or she can structure time so as to keep in touch with the feelings of staff nurses. This generally involves making rounds, holding open staff meetings, dealing directly with staff nurse committees, and occasionally getting involved in patient situations. As the nursing administrator displays caring behavior in meetings, conversations, and dealings with nurses, patients, families, and physicians, the caring norm begins to coalesce in the institution. As employees see and feel expressions of caring, the attitudes of caring are reproduced in patient situations.

Developing caring relationships with nursing managers and leaders also requires direct contact in which to display caring behaviors. As the nurse administrator makes rounds, he or she is able to interact with nurse managers on their own turf. Being alert to the atmosphere on the unit, talking to the staff, and visiting patients create opportunities to learn about the nurse manager's world. Allowing time to visit with the nurse manager on the nursing unit is often very productive. The manager, typically more open in a familiar environment, will be able to share successes and problems more readily.

In relation to nonmanagement nurse leaders (e.g. educators, clinical specialists, and quality assurance and discharge planning personnel), opportunities for caring interactions are facilitated by keeping up to date on their programs and taking a few minutes to interact with them informally whenever possible. In the case of all nurse managers and leaders, consulting with them individually when issues arise in their areas of expertise constitutes caring through validation of their sense of worth.

While we should encourage nurse administrators to develop caring relationships wherever possible in the organization, caring for their closest associates (assistant nursing directors and others reporting directly to the administrator) must be accorded top priority. In these relationships the nurse administrator must create time and opportunity to develop one-on-one caring. Those directly supervised become the significant others in the organizational setting. Setting up small group retreats and regular administrative meetings enhances cohesiveness and caring. In moments of private counseling, the nurse administrator should focus energy on the growth of the individual being counseled.

Openness

The fourth attribute contributing to caring in the administrative role is the development of personal values and behaviors that allow those cared for to risk being honest with the one who cares. This sets the stage for openness, which develops into trust and growth in the relationship. Being open is much more difficult than it sounds. Being open means being willing to disclose your own humanity, your unflattering thoughts as well as your noble ones, your hopes and your fears, your priorities and your problem areas. As others see the administrator more and more as a "real person," they are able to reveal themselves with some sense of safety. The attitude that must be exhibited is that openness leads to growth for both people in an interaction.

Rather than projecting the image that "no news is good news" (i.e. problems not expressed are not problems at all), the nurse administrator must foster open discussion of all issues. Problems that are identified at their early stages are almost always easier to deal with than those that have festered long.

The behaviors involved in openness include listening, soliciting comments, watching nonverbal communication cues, asking the right questions, and waiting patiently for answers. Another behavior that portrays openness is requesting feedback concerning all major changes. All identified issues must be carefully processed if obstacles to achieving change are to be overcome.

An important aspect of developing openness relates to the ways in which nurse administrators respond to feedback. If they express anger or alarm at negative or controversial comments, openness will be suppressed. If they express appreciation for the information provided and confidence about solving problems, people will be willing to continue to risk being open. Developing positive approaches to problem solving contributes greatly to enhanced caring behaviors. The attribute of openness is more than just a willingness to hear: it is a willingness to perceive, to empathize, and to respond. Noddings discusses the need to "apprehend the other's reality, feeling what he feels as nearly as possible. The one-caring is sufficiently engrossed in the other to listen to him and take pleasure or pain in what he recounts. The one cared-for sees the concern, delight, or interest in the eyes of the one-caring and feels her warmth in both verbal and body language" (1984, p. 19).

For nurse administrators, openness includes the ability to focus quickly and completely on the reality of many individuals and groups with whom they interact each day. Often the tendency is to split one's attention between the current interaction and the many other items needing attention, decisions, and actions.

Certain measures can be instituted to aid the nurse administrator. For example, meetings or appointments can be scheduled to end fifteen minutes before the next one is to begin. During each fifteen-minute break, having access to an efficient and personable secretary or administrative assistant is invaluable.

In addition to several short breaks whenever possible, the nurse administrator should schedule a period of time each day with a colleague who can provide caring for the nurse administrator. An opportunity to empty one's mind of the needs of others, to share concerns, to discuss common personal interests, and simply to enjoy not having to be a caregiver can be immensely rejuvenating.

Ability to Bring Out Potential

The last attribute that promotes caring behaviors is the ability to bring out potential in others. As several authors have pointed out, the outcome of a caring relationship is growth in the cared-for. This element has as its foundation the belief that people have abilities and talents that can be enhanced through the care of others. The person who would care for another must be able to search for these abilities and develop skills in encouraging the other to strive toward self-growth.

The arena of nursing administration offers many opportunities to enhance the growth of others. Recognizing these opportunities requires a deep appreciation for the potential of people around you. Some nurse administrators, threatened by the abilities of others, tend to put people down rather than build them up, so that their own needs for power and control are met. Other administrators view people in accordance with Hertzberg's (in Young and Hayne, 1988) "Theory X," as basically lazy and self-centered, thus requiring close control and strict rewards and punishment. The caring nurse administrator views people as valuable and is interested in helping them to develop to their full potential.

It is possible, given the basic belief in the potential of people, to develop particular skills that motivate others. Liberal use of positive feedback is very useful, particularly if used in conjunction with gentle honesty about areas where growth should occur. Inquiring about people's hopes, dreams, and goals for the future can make the nurse administrator alert to opportunities that may help others to meet individual goals.

Both publicly and privately the nurse administrator should always acknowledge the successes of staff nurses or nurse managers. During difficult times for a nurse manager (for example, conflicts between staff nurses on different shifts), the nursing administrator must remain accessible to the troubled manager and continue to follow up with him or her until the situation is resolved. Throughout the crisis, the nurse administrator must offer help and suggestions, and must also clearly communicate faith in the manager's ability to handle the problem.

When a project must be delegated, the nurse administrator should take time to assess who might be interested and able to handle it. Delegation is not only a way of redistributing workloads, but also a tool for allowing others to exhibit their potential through successful handling of special assignments. The person receiving the assignment must feel that the nurse administrator will trust and support his or her work and provide the freedom to grow through the experience.

Motivating others is basically the process of knowing people well enough to identify their potential, providing opportunities for their potential to be realized, and giving meaningful praise and rewards for jobs well done. The nurse administrator must always strive to convey faith in his or her people's potential. When one communicates a positive expectation that people can achieve great things, they usually do. Communication by the nursing administrator that people are expected, and will be assisted, to develop their full potential is a strong message of caring.

The Meaning of Caring

These five attributes—commitment, sense of self-worth, ability to prioritize, openness, and ability to bring out potential in others—enable the nurse administrator to direct caring behaviors toward the growth of others. The preferred definition of caring, then, is:

> An interactive commitment in which the one caring is able, through a strong self-concept, ordering of life activities, and openness to the needs of others, and the ability to motivate others, to enact caring behaviors that are directed toward the growth of the cared-for, be it an individual or group.

Caring is an ethic that affects all of life's relationships. It is a way of relating to people that involves special skills of openness and responsiveness to the needs of others. It is also a specific responsibility of the nurse administrator in his or her formal role as one who cares for nurses in an organization. Caring is both a philosophy and a milieu created in the organization for the purpose of encouraging caring relationships among staff members and between nurses and patients.

The responsibility of the nurse administrator in relation to caring is thus threefold:

1. to understand caring as philosophy and an ethic to be established by organizational processes and structures;

2. to develop skills related to caring behaviors that are utilized in formal relationships with individuals and groups;

3. to be alert and responsive to opportunities to participate in situations involving nurse managers, nurses, administrative colleagues, and patients or families who have specific needs that allow the nurse administrator to behave as a caring person.

The goals of caring are meaningful relationships and the growth of people in the organizational environment. Patients benefit by enhancement of the healing process, and employees benefit by finding added meaning and rewards in their work. While the pressures of the increasingly businesslike environment of health care continue to mount, the nurse administrator can have great impact by ensuring that the element of human caring remains an organizational priory.

References

Gaut, D. (1983). A theoretic description of caring as action. In Leininger, M., ed., *Care: The Essence of Nursing and Health*. Detroit: Wayne State University Press, pp. 27–44.

Leininger, M., ed. (1986). *Care: The Essence of Nursing and Health*. Detroit: Wayne State University Press.

Mayeroff, M. (1971). *On Caring*. New York: Barnes and Noble Books.

Miller, K. (1987). The human care perspective in nursing administration. *The Journal of Nursing Administration* 17 (2):10–12.

Noddings, N. (1984). *Caring: A Feminine Approach to Ethics and Moral Education*. Berkeley: University of California Press.

Ray, M. A. (1982). A philosophic analysis of caring within nursing. In Leininger, M., ed. *Caring: An Essential Human Need*. Detroit: Wayne State University Press, pp. 25–37.

Watson, J. (1985). *Human Science and Human Care*. Norwalk, CT: Appleton-Century-Crofts.

Young, L. C., and A. N. Hayne (1988). *Nursing Administration: From Concepts to Practice*. Philadelphia: W.B. Saunders.

CHAPTER FOUR

Organizational Theory

This chapter examines organizational theory. While some of the theory is anything but caring, it is our goal to see through Watson's (1985) "new lens" and try to apply caring to the organizational literature. Organizational theory is a huge body of literature; we will deal with the parts of it that have influenced my thinking about nursing administration. Other people may chose other parts of organizational theory, but they are not necessarily interested in the caring theory specifically. After a rather critical review of bureaucracy, I will introduce you to some of the more caring authors I have found.

No one can really say when organizations began. Jackson et al. (1986) view the history of organizations as originating thousands of years ago when people organized for protection, food gathering, and building shelters. These authors believe that humans have a tendency toward organizing—that it is a part of instinct and evolutionary growth. Certainly, humans seem to want to organize. We work in organizations, we worship in organizations, we play in organizations. Some people seem to be "joiners" more than others, but no one is totally uninfluenced by some organization. Our biggest forms of organization are governments, which have been around since recorded history. Certainly, there are good and bad things about organizations, but Jackson et al. remind us that in the establishment of organization, individuals must be willing to agree to the establishment and adherence to rules. By forming group goals and preventing chaos, each member has to perform certain functions and refrain from untoward behaviors that might be detrimental to the group. So, organizing is a "mixed bag." It can be very helpful, but it requires some loss of individual freedom. Morgan (1986) agrees with that premise and believes that the imposition of rules can lead to the diminishment of creativity and freedom for the soul. In health care, nurses' jobs vary in freedom and domination. Traditionally, hospital nursing has been very structured, and many nurses feel the sense of domination. Many hospitals are now experimenting with new structures that would give nurses more freedom in their jobs. Other job settings, such as home care, are less structured.

Marriner-Tomey (1988) wrote that organizing is establishing a formal structure that provides the coordination of resources to accomplish objectives and determine position qualifications and descriptions. She recognizes that there are both formal and informal organizations. The formal organization facilitates large-scale coordination. It is associated with subdivision of labor, specialization, rules and standards, and technical efficiency. The informal organization helps people meet personal needs and provides social control of behavior. Communication takes place in both the formal and informal organization, and the facts may not correlate with each other. The wise administrator pays attention to both parts of the organization.

It seems to me that nurses' informal organizations are particularly strong. That makes it imperative for the nurse administrator to find ways to tap into the informal communication system. I did this by knowing as many nurses as possible and making rounds on all shifts. One night, I walked up to a nurses' desk with the night supervisor. The nurse on duty, not knowing who I was, started complaining about the futility of nursing care plans. She was embarrassed when we were introduced, but I assured her that her opinion was valid to me. I never quite trusted care plans again, and I remembered how the staff nurses felt about them.

Historically, there have been many organizational theories, but the first one identified was the bureaucracy. Bureaucratic organizations were first defined around the early 1900s. This is when we saw the growth of factories, which were organized to improve productivity—making more goods by organizing the work. The world was changed by the efforts of the bureaucracy, but it had good and bad characteristics.

Aldridge (1979) sees bureaucratic organizations as technically superior for accomplishing complex tasks. Specialization limits each member to a subset of a task, and efficiency increases as members gain experience in their particular tasks. The problem with this division of labor is that, when a worker is assigned to do one task over and over and does not see their contribution to the end goal, their work feels very routine, boring, and dissatisfying. Visions come to mind of the old sweatshops where working conditions were deplorable. But not all bureaucracies were sweatshops; many were just efficient places to work, and employees were treated respectfully.

In the early 1900s, several organizational theorists defined organizations for the first time, and the organization they focused on was the bureaucracy. The bureaucracy was defined by Max Weber (1978), a German sociologist. He described the "ideal" organization as the bureaucracy. He recognized the good parts of the bureaucracy, but he also said that he was very concerned about what harm the bureaucracy could do to a society. In the past, most work was done by craftsmen (that is, a chair would be made by one person who would complete the task alone, and the chair was his creation). There was pride and a sense of accomplishment. In the new bureaucratic organization, one person might make the legs of the chair, someone else might make the back of the chair, and a third man may glue the chair together. What is lost is the sense of pride and ownership that the craftsman felt in creating the whole chair himself.

Nurses have been subjected to the bureaucracy, especially in hospitals. We organized our work into sets of tasks like other bureaucracies, and work became centered on accomplishing tasks, and the whole task of taking care of patients became fractured. Not only was this hard on the nurses, but patients also felt chopped up into parts and not treated as whole individuals.

Taylor (1978) was an early advocate of the bureaucracy. His work was devoted to further defining the bureaucracy and, in particular, he advocated the study of every task to determine the best (fastest) way to engineer work. This has happened in nursing in developing patient classification systems. The danger is in deciding who can do the various tasks. In our system, we used mostly RNs, and were able to keep away from saying such things as "all baths can be given by aides." We tallied up patient care hours, but we decided who would do the tasks according to our overall staffing policies. Taylor advocated five management principles:

1. Shift all responsibility for the organizing of work from the worker to the manager: managers do the thinking, workers implement tasks.

2. Use scientific methods to determine the most efficient way of doing a task, and specify to the worker the precise way to do the work.

3. Select the best person to perform the job designed.

4. Train the worker to do the work efficiently.

5. Monitor worker performance to ensure that appropriate work procedures are followed and that appropriate results are achieved.

Many other authors have written of the bureaucracy, and certain characteristics were repeated over and over. The bureaucracy was to be rule-oriented; there was to be a clear line of authority; bosses had the final say over everything; organizational charts were to be formulated to show clearly who was in charge of whom; discipline of employees was to be consistent to "keep every one in line"; there was to be a subordination of individual interests to general interests of the organization; conduct at work was to be formal and impersonal; initiative was to be rewarded; and employees were expected to be loyal to the organization. Taylor wrote about the potential problem of what he termed "soldiering," in which workers believed it was to their advantage to go slow. If one person did his work faster, there would be pressure from management for everyone to go faster, so everyone should go slow. Taylor was sometimes referred to as the enemy of the working man (Morgan, 1986). I believe this lack of trust is the atmosphere in many bureaucracies, and it has resulted in a "we versus they" attitude that does the organization no good in any way. It implies that people are basically lazy, and there is no emphasis on the worker feeling cared for.

The bureaucracy worked very well for certain tasks and at certain times. As long as nothing changed, the bureaucracy did a marvelous job of improving the output of goods. The standard of living in the industrialized world improved enormously. Jobs were created so that people had money to buy the manufactured goods, and it affected society in a positive way. Even organizations that did not produce goods adopted the model of the bureaucracy. Service organizations, such as hospitals, organized bureaucratically, but with difficulty. As the years went by, problems developed that these organizations could not handle.

Bureaucracies had two particular flaws. The first flaw was that the bureaucracy could not accommodate quickly to change. People were comfortable in their well-defined jobs, but what the routinization had taken away was the employees' being able to think for themselves. And, with the monstrously complex organizational structure, it was almost impossible to get decisions made quickly.

The second fatal flaw of the bureaucracy was that it did not take into account the needs of the nonmanagement employees. The employees were tired of feeling like they could not think, and they were tired of not having any say over how their lives were organized. They got tired of doing work that seemed meaningless because they could not see the connection between their work and an end product they could feel proud of. Nurses were relegated to be bath nurses, medication nurses, and desk nurses. They were tired of the isolation where everyone focused on their own task and no one felt a sense of comradery. They got tired of rules that rarely made sense in the real work environment, and they got tired of people—who rarely knew as much about the work as they did—telling them what to do. I am sure that these feelings are not unknown by nurses who have worked very long. In fact, there are still health care organizations where nurses feel very dominated by their organizations. Nurses are asked to be caring to patients, but the bureaucracy is not caring to them.

Another example of our leftover bureaucracy is apparent when organizational change occurs. Particularly if financial crises occur, the organization shuts down its "participative model," and distressed managers emerge from closed-door meetings where decisions revert to rigid bureaucracy. Employees are told (not asked) to do more with less, and the wealth of employee ideas is rarely sought out, let alone implemented.

Why spend so much time describing an old organizational model? Because, in nursing and health care, it has not gone away. Oh, we make change after change, thinking that we are moving in the right direction. Then, along comes the Joint Commission of Accreditation of Health Care Organizations, and we drag out the policy and procedure books, we brush off the organizational chart, and we present ourselves as the perfect bureaucracy. Many hours are spent on updating policies and on teaching the nurses the right answers to possible questions. Everything is cleaned, and the workday clutter is hidden in any corner. The acuity system and nursing care plans are embellished. We try often to clean up a four-year mess in a four-week binge.

When I was a staff nurse in an emergency room, things were quite bureaucratized. We had thick policy and procedure books, and the nurse–doctor relationship was very hierarchical—nurses were never to question doctors. One night, a patient came in to our emergency room not feeling well. He said he had a heaviness in his chest, but not really any pain. His only pain was in his right elbow, and his vital signs were fine. His respirations were slightly labored and he was very anxious. I called his doctor, who told me to put him in an ambulance and send him to another hospital. I said I was uneasy about that, and asked if the emergency room doctor could see him. He said no, to just send him. I found myself up against a bureaucratic wall. I was to do what was ordered, yet I felt that it was not safe to send him. I decided to stall for a while. I remember telling the patient that his doctor wanted him transferred, but that I wanted to watch him for awhile. I went to the nursing station and tried to talk the emergency room doctor into seeing the patient. He was hesitant because of his hierarchical boundaries. While we were talking, I looked over at the patient and saw that he was seizing and then he collapsed into cardiac arrest. Fortunately, the patient was revived, and no one could give me much grief about it, but I remember feeling very frustrated that I had to agonize over using my own judgment. I think the only thanks I got was from the patient when he came back to see us in a couple of months. Since we were working in a very bureaucratic organization, the only formal action taken was to write another policy saying that the nurses could ask the emergency room doctor to see anyone that the nurse felt uneasy about transporting. If I had known about caring at the time, I would have recognized that I was using my intuitive judgment, and I would have trusted it. I would have acknowledged my expertness and ability to judge the whole of the situation. The organization would have recognized my good judgment, and I would have received positive feedback from my supervisor.

Clearly, up to this point, there is very little caring theory in organizational theory. The emphasis has been on what was best for the organization, not the people in them. However, in the 1950s and 1960s, organizational theory took a drastic turn. It began with the Hawthorn studies, which were originally studying the effects of changing levels of light in work areas. The researchers were surprised to find that output increased in both the areas where more light was introduced and in the control group, which had changed nothing. The conclusion was that just the attention given to the groups by being in the study changed the worker's behavior. The human-relations movement began. Instead of focusing on the work, theorists began focusing on the employees. Maslow (in Marriner-Tomey, 1988) identified his famous "hierarchy of needs," which told of workers needs for things other than a paycheck. His hierarchy started at the bottom with physiological needs, followed by needs for safety, needs for social interaction, needs for self-esteem, and, at the top, the personal needs to feel self-actualized (to be at their best in their world).

Nurses have used Maslow's hierarchy of needs, not only in relationship to their own needs as employees, but also in defining the needs of their patients. Trying to meet patients' needs is part of caring, as is meeting employees' needs. This type of theory (human-relations) is more caring because it attends to personal needs. Organizations that can understand that they need to meet employees' needs so that employees can meet consumers' needs have begun to understand caring in relation to organizations.

Hertzberg (in Young and Hayne, 1988) identified what things in the workplace were "dissatisfiers" and which were "satisfiers." The dissatisfiers were things like salary and benefits, and when they were not perceived as appropriate, the employees felt dissatisfied. However, when these things were attended to properly, the employees were not necessarily satisfied. The satisfiers were related to the work itself, such as work autonomy, job content, and being able to be creative in their work. Nurses, like most employees, need to feel fulfilled in their work.

McGreggor (in Young and Hayne, 1988) wrote about how there are two ways of looking at people: one, as basically lazy thus needing prodding and discipline at work, and two, as basically good and ambitious and wanting to work their best if given the chance. Bureaucracies see employees as basically lazy, while caring organizations see employees as trying to do their best.

Likert (in Marriner-Tomey 1988) wrote that there are four types of management systems: 1. exploitive-authoritative; 2. benevolent-authoritarian; 3. consultative; and 4. participatory. While he believes there are different settings where each type may be used, he prefers the participative style where superiors have complete confidence in their subordinates, open communication is present, and goals are set at all levels in the organization. Likert's participative model has been the goal of many nursing organizations. I used the model to improve communications and open up the organization so that nurses felt autonomous and valued in our hospital. I now see this model as a useful way to start a caring process in organizations because caring depends on communication and openness.

Human relations departments were organized during the 1960s and 1970s, and much attention was given to job design and employee job satisfaction. Morgan (1986) is skeptical of such management moves, as he says they offered the possibility of motivating employees through "higher level" needs without paying them more. This may be true, but it was a step in the right direction to attend to employees' higher level needs.

Some authors created "'sociotechnical' systems" where jobs and technology were matched. Woodward (1978) found in her studies that technical methods were the most important factor in determining organizational structure. For organizations that make defined, simple products, bureaucracies work well because the focus is on defining tasks to maximize output. For more complex organizations, especially if they have to respond to environmental changes, the structure needs to be more differential and more open to communication from employee to manager and vise-versa.

Hospitals are among the most complex of organizations. The product varies with every patient, and technical change is constant. In these systems, it is important to have structures where communication is ongoing and employees can make their own decisions when necessary. The caring theory calls for open communication and feelings of connectedness that can only be well established with organizational structures which encourage people to think and act in different ways depending on each patient's needs.

The next group of theories focused on systems theory, which was developed by Ludwig von Bertalanffy (as discussed in Morgan, 1986). Morgan wrote, "The systems approach builds on the principle that organizations, like organisms, are 'open' to their environment and must achieve an appropriate relation with that environment if they are to survive" Morgan (1986, p. 44) and Boulding (1978) described systems at the frameworks level, the clockworks level, the thermostat level, the cell level, the plant level, the animal level, the human level, the social organization level, and the transcendental systems level. Each level incorporates all those below it, and analysis can be applied at various levels. In open systems, the emphasis is on the environment, scanning and sensing changes related to your organization. Each system is viewed as interrelated with subsystems and supersystems, and the task is to establish congruencies between different systems. Systems theory is used by nurses as they assess patients, as well as when they assess the organization. It is caring in that it looks at relationships and connections.

Another group of theories derive from the contingency theorists. Authors such as Burns and Stalker and Lawerence and Lorsh (in Morgan, 1986) wrote about the relationship between leaders and their organizations. These theories contend that there is no one best way of organizing. In contingency theory, the manager is expected to modify leadership style depending on the type of organization and the situation at hand. It makes sense, but it may confuse everyone to not be able to count on consistent actions from their managers. At its best, contingency theory may be able to move the organization toward a flexible style referred to as "adhocracy," which is temporary by design. Leaders organize work groups to work on a particular issue and then change the design when the task changes. Such organizational structures can be very confusing, but work reasonably well in organizations undergoing constant change. Many adhocracies utilize a "matrix organization." Matrix forms are team-driven and encourage flexible, innovative, and adaptive behavior. Unfortunately, they become very confusing to work in, and much time can be wasted trying to get the communications where they need to be.

Nursing organizations can use many of these types of structures. To coincide with the caring theory, they need to be structures that work for nurses. Nursing varies in different specialties, though, and the nurse manager should be able to help decide on the structure of the nursing unit. In the emergency department, a more autocratic leadership style may be appropriate. Medical and rehabilitation units need to be more flexible so that caregivers have the latitude to make decisions on their own. During cardiac arrests, someone needs to be barking out orders; during a team conference, everyone deserves time and openness to express themselves. Management is an art, and the best skill a manager can develop is to read people and situations so that they can be handled appropriately.

Often, nursing divisions are far ahead of the organization as a whole at moving beyond the bureaucracy. But it is hard to hang on to our collegial ideals when the hospital administrators try to take control and meet organizational stresses by themselves. Even many nursing administrators revert to hierarchical control during events such as layoffs or budget crunches. This creates problems, because, if the manager exerts bureaucratic control just once, the staff will lose trust in the participation process that was built up over a long time period. Even though the nursing administrator cannot share everything with staff, explanations of decisions and honest assessments of where the organization is going are important to nurses throughout the organization.

Least we be too hard on ourselves, it is important to look at other industries in our country. Certainly, health care is not the only industry reverting to bureaucratic organization models. Large corporations are cutting staff, merging into huge conglomerates, and increasing productivity in any way possible. There are not a whole lot of nonbureaucratic organizations in Americans' corporate reality. One must ask, if there are nonbureaucratic theories around, why are our organizations still so bureaucratic and uncaring? It is probably because it is hard to leave the bureaucracy behind. Using more open systems is a time-consuming and tiring thing. Even though we know that the bureaucracy has its problems, it is sometimes tempting to sit back and blast out orders.

As we begin to look at some of the newer organizational structures, let us keep an eye out for caring concepts. Let's also think about how some of the newer organizational theories could be implemented in our real-life organizations. Some of you readers will be encouraged and some will be discouraged. But, we should remember that organizational theorists have been calling for more flexible, people-oriented organizational models for nearly forty years. Sometimes I wonder if the theorists just have their heads in the clouds—not seeing or writing about reality. Then I think, what if they did not write idealistic and futuristic ideas? Deep down, I feel that things improve slowly, as on a roller coaster ride—slowly at first and later faster. If we can't create an ideal for the future, we will certainly never get there! So, let us examine a few of the newest theorists and see if we can find some caring in their ideas.

In the 1970s and 1980s new organizational authors emerged, and some of their books became immensely popular. A dominate series has been the *Megatrends* books. In the first *Megatrends*, Naisbitt (1982) defined ten trends that he thought were going to change the world in general and organizations in particular. In the next book, *Megatrends 2000*, Naisbitt and Aburdene (1990) said that the 1980s were the decade when economics became more important than ideologies. They predicted that the 1990s will also be a period of economic prosperity. These authors recognized that foreign investments were on the rise, and that people feel uneasy about foreigners taking over our country. But they contend that no country is better positioned than the United States because we have a fantastic human resource mix of well-educated, skilled information workers.

I am not too sure that these facts could be confirmed in the mid-1990s. With the tremendous drop in employment, many of our bright, skilled workers are beating the pavement looking for jobs. Naisbitt and Aburdene see a need for new kinds of management for the twenty-first century. They call for leaders that think long term, affirm values, achieve unity, inspire commitment, and empower people by sharing authority. This is very hard to do if the organization is only looking for a hefty bottom line. Naisbitt and Auburdene believe that the primary challenge of leadership in the 1990s is to encourage the new, better-educated worker to be more entrepreneurial, self-managing, and oriented toward lifelong learning. They believe that the primary principle of the organization has shifted, from management in order to control a business to leadership in order to bring out the best in people and to respond quickly to change. Naisbitt and Aburdene say that the great unifying theme at the conclusion of the twentieth century is the triumph of the individual. They believe that the most exciting breakthroughs will occur not because of technology but of an expanding concept of what it means to be human.

Naisbitt and Auburdene certainly paint a rosy picture of the years ahead, yet we are over one-half of the way there, and I do not feel we are attaining very much. I sense very little caring in corporate America, and I think few organizations are focusing on the expanding concept of the individual. But let's take a look at the megatrends they defined for the twenty-first century. They were:

1. The Booming Global Economy of the 1990s.
2. A Renaissance of the Arts.
3. The Emergence of Free-Market Socialism.
4. Global Lifestyles and Cultural Nationalism.

A Caring Approach in Nursing Administration

5. The Privatization of the Welfare State.
6. The Rise of the Pacific Rim.
7. The Decade of Woman in Leadership.
8. The Age of Biology.
9. The Religious Revival of the New Millennium.
10. The Triumph of the Individual.

(Naisbitt and Auburdene 1990, p. 13)

One could argue for hours about whether these megatrends are emerging, but it is clear that these organizational theorists have an expansionary sense of the future. The booming global economy is happening, but I don't see a renaissance of the arts or the emergence of free-market socialism. Certainly the rise of the Pacific Rim area is taking place and women are doing better in business. I guess what I get from this book is a feeling of positive excitement. In nursing, I think that the trends are particularly positive. For example, Watson's caring theory calls for more attention to be placed on the arts. Nurses are discovering that music, touch, and relaxation are helping to allay fears and anxieties in patients. Nursing is also encouraging the understanding of various cultures when taking care of patients. We are seeing the emergence of women in nursing and health care leadership. Caring certainly validates the importance of the spiritual aspect in nurses and their patients, and it validates the extreme importance of individuals.

Another book of our time that became very popular in organizational circles was *In Search of Excellence* (Peters and Waterman, 1982). These authors studied successful organizations to identify what characteristics made them successful. The qualities, along with my loose interruption of their applications to nursing, are:

1. "A bias for action."—This quality means don't study things to death. In nursing, it means taking action for patients even if there are obstacles. In administration it means taking action sometimes even without all the data you would like.

2. "Close to the customer."—This is the cornerstone of nursing. It means putting patients needs first every time. It means, to these authors, that you get information from customers before and after developing your product. I think this is something nursing could do much more of. Too often *we* decide what we think is best, rather

than asking the patient what they think they need. We should include families in our planning about patients. We should also get feedback (usually in the form of questionnaires or interviews) from patients regularly.

3. "Autonomy and entrepreneurship."— This refers to letting employees have the authority to make decisions about their work, and encouraging them to think of new services. It also refers to the whole organization having a spirit of innovation.

4. "Productivity through people."—Respect your employees and help them to find ways to improve their productivity. So many times when I speak to nurses, they have wonderful ideas that would cut costs, but it seems impossible to implement them. Recently, a nurse suggested letting people bring their medications from home and take them themselves. Of course the pharmacy had a fit, but we have to begin to look at things with a more open approach to do the cost-cutting ahead.

5. "Hands-on, values driven."—Peters and Waterman believe in managers that get out and see employees in their setting, not in the administrator's office. For nursing administrators, it means going into patients' rooms and into nurses' stations. Their agenda should always be to encourage the implementation of the values of caring.

6. "Stick to the knitting."—Many companies have diversified, including hospitals that have bought everything from clinics to real estate. Perhaps Peters and Waterman were right—many companies are selling off unrelated businesses and getting back to what they do best. The *Wall Street Journal* recently had an article about companies trimming alternative businesses to get back to their original business. Hospitals are also getting rid of unrelated businesses.

7. "Simple form, lean staff."—These authors are opposed to long, confusing organizational charts. They advocate a streamlined business where only necessary people are hired. In nursing, that is currently reflected in reevaluating educators and clinical nurse specialists. Each job will need to show how it is of value to the primary goal of patient care.

8. "Simultaneous loose-tight properties."—This is my personal favorite. To me it means having a few absolute values that you expect nurses to adhere to, and then giving them all kinds of room to decide how to meet those values.

Peters and Waterman found that one of the most basic properties in successful companies was the respect they had for people—both their customers and their staff. This book is fairly dated now, but I included it because I think it has "worn well." The authors have written other books, but I still come back to this one. Perhaps it is also because a study was done in nursing using the principles of *In Search of Excellence*. Kramer and Schmalenberg (1988) did a restudy of the Magnet Hospitals in 1988 and compared Peters and Waterman's principles to the operation of the magnet hospitals. They found a great deal of congruency. I found great hope for caring when I read this book. The principles are implementable and lead to the goal of meeting the needs of people along with the needs of the organization.

Peters (1992) of Peters and Waterman wrote another book called *Liberation Management* in which he posits that it is time to "blow up" the huge conglomerates in favor of many small working units with minimal central control. This includes getting rid of middle-managers and functional departments and doing the work in project teams that have the autonomy to do business themselves. He says that we must attempt to get close to the market, staying small enough to shift focus fast. He advocates "putting the zanies in charge" (p. 14), and unleashing the power to the subordinate units. In his view, most managers have added negative value to corporations. There should be no need for anyone to get permission from anyone "above" them—decisions should rest with the work units. He likes the idea of adhocracies where holding companies coordinate the work of numerous temporary work units—phasing in and out of existence according to the rate of change. In order to empower people, Peters suggests that you make it so you have way too many people to manage, so they will figure out how to work without close supervision. Likewise, he suggests that the project teams that are held responsible for results should be a little understaffed. This may work in some settings, but I have witnessed one organization that slashed its administrative system and formed working committees, and the result was chaos. While it would seem ideal to not have such organizational structures, most organizations need some structure and pointed decision making.

Peters focuses specifically on hospitals in one area of his book. He said that, for every dollar hospitals spend directly on patient care, they spend three or four dollars waiting for it to happen, arranging to do it, and writing it down.

He referenced J. Philip Lathrop in the July/August 1991 issue of *Healthcare Forum Journal,* who reported about one hospital where they implemented "care pairs" and "patient-focused hospital." Basically, in the past, the health care industry made thousands of sound decisions that now add up to a mess. For example, we have a system where we have convinced ourselves and our patients that a two-hour process of getting a routine x-ray is a good system. We have a system where more than half the lab tests are ordered "stat" just to get the results in a fairly good time. We have a preoccupation with specialization that results in five-minute EKGs taking an hour to schedule, document, and transport. We have specialists with set job descriptions that are so restricted that no one will do anything out of their job specifications. There is an infrastructure where clerks and secretaries outnumber the inpatients, and the number of department heads number sixty to a hundred people.

In Peters's study hospital, the cross-trained care-givers can provide 80 to 90 percent of the needs of four to seven patients. The care pairs "own" their patients, maintaining a continuity for patients. Ancillary services were performed for the convenience of patients and doctors, and documentation now takes less than thirty minutes per care-giver per day. Quality is enhanced so that auditing the process of care is not needed, and 15 to 20 percent sustainable reductions in personnel are possible.

The results of this program have been that turnaround time for routine tests dropped from 157 minutes to 48 minutes, the care-givers spend twice the time with patients, there are fewer falls and medication errors, and soaring satisfaction levels.

This is an exciting example of a very creative nursing care delivery systems change. It would be interesting to hear what the nurses have to say about it. Most certainly, nurses will be expected to do some nonnursing chores, which is always frustrating, but I like the idea of small working units that operate on their own. I think many nursing departments have already done that as units have become more autonomous. The idea of small work groups that come together for one defined purpose and then go away could be a description of patient care conferences. The idea of "care pairs" leads to more continuity in who takes care of the patient, and this allows time for the development of caring relationships between nurses and patients.

Another author that has advocated some similar ideas is Kantor (1983), who wrote in *Change Masters* that organizations need to promote a climate of success and a culture of pride. Different jobs need to be more connected so that people feel they belong to a meaningful enterprise. Movement away from the rigid bureaucracy can increase creativity and response to changes, and people feel more pride in the company as they work together on teams or projects. As pride increases, employees typically achieve greater productivity and work satisfaction. Perhaps it is not surprising that this author is a woman (not that they are *all* caring), and her work certainly fits with the caring theory. It encourages the connectedness and meaning that Watson writes about and leads to pride in excellent patient care.

Another contemporary author about organizations is Gareth Morgan. He wrote *Images of Organizations,* in which he describes bureaucracies as "organizations as machines." He believes that bureaucracies work well under conditions where machines work well—when there is a straightforward task and the environment is stable. He sees the limits of bureaucracies as:

1. having great difficulty in adapting to changing circumstances;

2. resulting in mindless and unquestioning behavior;

3. allowing the organizational task to take precedence over the broader goals the organization was designed for; and

4. having a dehumanizing effect upon employees, especially those at the lower levels.

Morgan writes, "Defining work responsibilities in a clear-cut manner has the advantage of letting everyone know what is expected of them. . . . [but] This institutionalized passivity and dependency can even lead people to make and justify deliberate mistakes on the premise that they're obeying orders" (Morgan 1986, p. 36).

Morgan suggests other metaphors (besides machines) to explore organizations. For example, he wrote about organizations as organisms—

living systems, existing in a wider environment on which they depend for the satisfaction of various needs. This metaphor has helped theorists to identify and study different organizational needs as "open systems." Organizations can be seen as adapting organisms that respond to environmental change. Morgan suggests other metaphors such as organizations as brains, as cultures, as political systems, as psychic prisons, as flux and transformation, or as instruments of domination. The image of organizations as brains is an interesting one for nursing organizations. The brain metaphor encourages the values of openness and reflectivity that accepts errors and uncertainty. It encourages analysis and solution of complex problems by exploring different options. The key to the brain is connectivity and self-organization.

If a nursing organization used the brain metaphor, there would be a view of the whole, not just the parts, and the emphasis would be on connecting the parts of the organization to make a meaningful whole. These ideas are consistent with Benner's and Watson's conception of caring, where emphasis is on heath as wholeness. Each of the metaphors presents a very different view of organizations. They each have strengths and weaknesses, but one of the main reasons to study metaphors is to go beyond thinking of organizations in one rigid way—as bureaucratic machines.

In Morgan's 1993 book, *Imaginization,* he takes the idea of metaphors a little further. He advocates organizations thinking up their own metaphors to learn more about how they feel about their organizations. He describes experiments where major players in the organization go away for a "retreat." The facilitator begins by giving some examples of different metaphors, and then he/she asks the employees to make up their own metaphors of how they see their organizations at work. The different metaphors are shared with all participants, and then the group tries to negotiate to a metaphor they can all agree on. From here, free discussions occur about how the organization can be improved.

Morgan's method defines "imaginization" as infusing the process of organizing with a spirit of imagination that takes us beyond bureaucratic bosses to find creative ways of organizing and managing that allow us to use new images and ideas. It is a means of empowering people to trust themselves and find new roles in our changing organizations.

Morgan's books have been some of my favorites because they are readable and offer very creative ideas about new ways of thinking about

A Caring Approach in Nursing Administration

organizations. I think they can be very useful to nurse administrators who need some outside ideas. His books all have a creative and people-oriented approach to them, and I think they can help to think up new ways to apply and enhance the caring approach. In my work as a nursing administrator, I used retreats in a very positive way. Our leadership group had one annually, and many of the nursing units had them also. It is very helpful to get out the work setting where you aren't listening for a page or worrying about whether someone is taking care of your patients. In the retreats, we did goal setting, bonding, and problem solving. I was never creative enough to think up a method such as Morgan's metaphors, but I think it would be an excellent way to start creative thinking.

Another innovative way to look at organizations is to view them as having life cycles. The young organization typically spends all its time and all its energy making its products or services. As the organization matures, competition and outside pressures grow, and the organization finds itself spending more resources on politics, administration, legal protection, and planning ways to defend itself. As the organization reaches old age, sometimes the bulk of its resources are used to defend itself and fight off change. Lodahl and Mitchell (1980) define positive maturity in organizations as the ability to reproduce its values and ideals—to boldly direct its life-cycle realities and become regenerative as an organization of the future as well as the past. They discuss the concept of organizational drift, where a gap develops between the founder's ideals and intentions and the enacted organization. A successful organization is one that is able to ensure consensus of values and ideals across generations of workers. The organizational pioneers must create symbolic language, ritual, and organizational structures that perpetuate the organization's mission. Members are recruited who believe in the organization's ideals, and if the structure hinders the ideology, it is replaced. The organization is a success to the degree that it exhibits authenticity, functionality, feasibility, and employee commitment across generations.

The organizational life-cycle theory is very important to nursing. Our founders clearly established a caring focus in nursing. We have, I think, successfully perpetuated our caring values regardless of the organizational structure or circumstance. The question is, "Can we continue to practice caring when our industry (health care) reaches the maturity level of old age, where the outside enemy uses more of our energy than the central effort of caring?" That will be our central challenge, in my view, in the next decade of health care.

Another author I want to focus on is W. Edwards Deming. I must confess that after reading several articles written by and about him, I remain a little puzzled about just what his philosophy includes. I know that Deming was originally a statistician who went to Japan after World War II to help rebuild the Japanese manufacturing base. He is known in Japan as a great thinker about organizations, and the Japanese feel they owe much of their organizational success to his leadership. In America, Deming has just "caught on" in the past few years.

Lawton (1993) describes Deming's philosophy as based on the principle of total quality management. He believes that the goal should not be to test small quantities of goods for quality, but that the goal is to work continually on the system to make sure that every item produced is of high quality. He believes that there are no bad people, just bad systems, so there should be constant improvements in systems. To do that, the ideas for the improvements usually come from production employees, so the company should treat its people as its most valuable resource. I agree with focusing on systems' improvements, but I think there can be people-problems that must be addressed along with the systems' problems.

Deming does not agree with the American passions of independence and competition. Rather, he stresses the ideas of cooperation and interdependence (which are also found in the caring literature). He believes that people have lots of intrinsic motivation to do their best work, and this translates into organizational success. He says that cooperation is driven by the realization that my success is tied to yours. He would do away with the competitiveness among employees and treat them all the same. Gillem (1988) wrote about Deming's ideas as they apply to hospitals. He identified fourteen key points:

1. "Create constancy of purpose for service improvement."— concern should be for long-term, not short-term goals. Communicate constancy of purpose to all employees.

2. "Adopt the new philosophy."—that it is possible for things to be done right the first time. Do not look for errors at the end of production, but expect things to be done right the first time.

3. "Cease dependence on inspection to achieve quality."—particularly in a hospital, where there is no room for error. Focus attention on improving the entire process or system of care.

4. "End the practice of rewarding business on price alone. Make partners out of vendors." (This goal is very important in hospitals. For example, if you buy equipment because of price alone, you might really get burned if it does not work or requires a lot of special training to use.)

5. "Constantly improve every process for planning, production, and service." Gillem says that the health care industry can no longer solicit suggestions from workers and then do nothing about them.

6. "Institute training and retraining on the job."—quality will improve as workers learn to collect and use information to guide their improvement efforts.

7. "Institute leadership for system improvement."—the manager must be the leader for the improvement of the system's performance.

8. "Drive out fear."—if workers are afraid of making improvements or making suggestions for improvements they will not make them.

9. "Break down barriers between staff areas."—health care is full of barriers between different types of providers. We must learn not to complain about other's jobs, but work to understand them. This is an area that nurses have been slow to accept. But the nurse is in the pivotal position to coordinate services. In the past, "multidisciplinary" meant everybody got referred to every department we could think of, but in the cost-conscious 1990s, nurses will be asked to minimize referrals to only the ones that are likely to make a big difference. Nurses, while continuing to cooperate with other providers, will have a large responsibility to minimize services because of costs.

10. "Eliminate slogans, exhortations, and targets for the work force." They are an insult.

11. "Eliminate numerical quotas for the work force and numerical goads for the management." If the initial focus in on quantity, quality will suffer.

12. "Remove barriers to pride of workmanship." "Management behavior that urges employees to more effectively work together is far more important than behavior that promotes individual performances" (p. 77).

13. "Institute a vigorous program of education and self-improvement for everyone." Quality begins and ends with education.

14. "Put everyone to work on the transformation." Everyone is needed to make it happen.

Deming's work makes sense, but parts of it are radically different than the typical management in America. We are so absorbed in competition that the idea of doing away with performance appraisals and merit raises is very foreign to us. Considering cooperation as more important than competition is not the American way. Come to think of it, though, I cannot think of very many times when performance appraisals were of help and not miserable for the employee and the supervisor. Nursing is by nature more cooperative than some health care providers, because we have to get along with everyone to get things done. Maybe Deming has something good to say to us, after all.

The weaknesses I see in Deming's work are that it is still leader-driven and there is emphasis on conforming to preset job goals and standards. There seems to be little emphasis on creativity, experience, and intuition. Deming's Quality Improvement Model still retains a fairly tight bureaucratic control, though he emphasizes employee involvement in defining the job requirements. There is an emphasis on reducing variance and involving customers in defining organizational goals. In patient care settings, quality is not always totally understood or recognized by patients, but I do agree that we should include them in our planning. Deming also seems to assume that decreased costs result in increased quality, which is not necessarily so. In health care, technical innovation makes it very hard to decrease costs. This sets up the problem of cutting staff, who do the basic work of patient care, in order to keep up with other hospitals' technology. All the technology may make it easier to decrease physical disease, but we have established that all cure with no care is not desirable. Cost cutting can be very deleterious to caring if we don't keep patient care providers in such numbers that care can be delivered optimally.

Several other authors have written important organizational books in the past few years. Senge (1990) wrote *The Fifth Discipline,* in which the focus is on systems thinking. This author writes that vision is the key to organizational success, but the leader has to be able to make the vision everybody's vision, not just the leader's vision. This is particularly important in nursing. If the leader is the only one tuned in to a caring value system, it will not succeed in the organizational system. The role of the leader is to teach the vision and be open to changing the vision as it evolves. He describes the "learning organization," where people continually expand their capacity to create the results they truly desire. In the learning organization, new and expansive patterns of learning are nurtured, and people are encouraged to learn together. In caring, there is always more to learn—about yourself and about patients and employees. Nurses want more than anything to take care of patients in the best way they know how. The result they desire is caring, for themselves and for their patients.

Senge also wrote about "metanoia," which is a work experience where there is a great team feeling, and the people have the feeling of being engaged in something bigger than themselves. He says that business is the locus of innovation in our society because it has the freedom to experiment and a clear bottom for evaluation. His emphasis is on people—what they can create and the immense satisfaction that can be achieved in the right organizational milieu. He also stresses building shared visions and team learning where people dialogue, think together, and discover new insights. The team IQ is higher than the individual IQ.

When I worked in the emergency room, there was a sense of the metanoia of which Senge speaks. When we accomplished a successful resuscitation, we felt "high." But there was also the sense of accomplishment in caring for a baby with a fever as well. I remember all the New year's Eve nights when we never would have made it if it were not for the sense of metanoia that came from working with a well-run team. When I became an administrator, I didn't expect to feel this way again. But as we established a new administration team and started working on primary nursing and participative management (which I now understand was my way of being a caring administrator), we again felt the immense satisfaction of our collective IQ being more than our individual IQs. We worked to establish an environment where nurses felt as cared for as we wanted them to care for patients.

Senge's laws of the "fifth discipline" are:

1. Today's problems come from yesterday's solutions.
2. The harder you push, the harder the system pushes back.
3. Behavior grows better before it grows worse.
4. The easy way out usually leads back in.
5. The cure can be worse than the disease.
6. Faster is slower.
7. Cause and effect are not closely related in time and space.
8. Small changes can produce big results, but the areas of highest leverage are often the least obvious.
9. You can have your cake and eat it too—but not all at once.
10. Dividing an elephant in half does not produce two small elephants.
11. There is no blame.   (Senge, 1990, pp. 57–67)

These laws can be humorous, but they are saying that you must be open to new things, don't get too caught up with yourself, and let some problems take care of themselves. As an administrator, I know there is a lot of wisdom in his words. Senge's book is complex and not easy to read, but it contains ideas consistent with our other people-oriented books and with using a caring ethic in business. It emphasizes values and people. Nursing is a lifelong learning job, so the idea of a learning organization is a good one. It emphasizes leaders who can bring out the best in people instead of bossing them. It is consistent with a caring focus.

Kotter (1990) wrote about leadership as a force for change. He emphasizes the difference between leaders and managers (which I have used interchangeably). He sees management as the function of creating order and consistency. He says that management is what we have had the last 100 years. Leadership, on the other hand, is the process of creating movement. He says that a good organization needs both good managers and good leaders, but that most organizations have an abundance of good managers and very few good leaders. The functions according to Kotter of the leader are: 1. direction setting; 2. getting people aligned with the direction; and 3. motivate and inspire. Kotter and Senge write about how important it is to have employees involved in defining goals and values for the organization. Then the goals are everyone's, not just something that comes down from on high. Kotter says that a good leader is one who can move people to a place in which both they and those who depend on them are genuinely better off without trampling upon the rights of others.

He believes that a good leader is a complex product of heredity, early life experiences, important career events, and the culture of their current organization. He does not go so far as to say that leaders are born, not educated, but he said that the four attributes of a good leader are 1. intelligence; 2. drive; 3. mental health; and 4. integrity. Kotter wrote that the ultimate act of leadership in an organization is creating a leadership-oriented culture that continues after the creator has gone.

Kotter's writings are also consistent with caring as they encourage leaders to be connected and understanding of their employee's needs and desires. I agree with Kotter that we have more good managers than we do leaders, and this is a time in health care when we desperately need leaders. Nursing leaders need to align the nurses with the caring mission, and that must be done delicately. Sometimes I think leaders just push too hard and feel like they have to have all the answers, rather than sitting back and working *with* everyone around them.

Badaracco and Ellsworth (1989) wrote *Leadership and the Quest for Integrity.* They defined integrity as consistency between what a manager believes, how a manager behaves, and what the manager's aspiration is for his/her organization. These authors define five management dilemmas:

1. Tension between a general, flexible, open-end approach vs. a precise, clear approach.

2. Tension between top-down and bottom-up approach.

3. Conflict between substance and process.

4. Confrontation vs. compromise.

5. Tension between tangibles and intangibles.

They believe that all of these approaches are appropriate at different times. They lean toward the first approaches in the dilemmas, but reserve the option of using the second approach when necessary. Basically, they believe in participatory organizations, but they feel strongly that leaders need to maintain overall control and accountability. Badarocco and Ellsworth describe three types of managers: 1. political leadership; 2. directive leadership; and 3. values-driven leadership. While there may be occasions for using the first two, values-driven leadership is preferred. The values-driven leader shapes an organization so that its values, norms, and ideals appeal strongly to its individual members while at the same time making the company a strong competitor. This means being clear and precise, and confronting conflicts directly. It means encouraging bottom-up influence while retaining the ability to get directly involved. Badarocco and Ellsworth write somewhat negatively about situational management or contingency management. In these styles, the leader changes styles according to what is going on at the time. They believe that, to be most effective, managers should avoid these styles. Instead, they should strive to be consistent in situations and their behavior should be consistent with their personalities, beliefs, and judgments. Management should approach the situations they face with a specific set of predispositions or prejudices so that everyone in the organization will see a consistency in the managers' behavior. This involves being preoccupied with substance, not process, and making persistent efforts to help intangibles overcome the tyranny of the tangible. The leader has two responsibilities: 1. infuse the company with a purpose, and 2. create an environment where employees are allowed to solve problems and create opportunities with deep personal commitment.

> In the final analysis, the power of executive leadership rests not so much on the personality of the individual as on the power of the ideas, purposes, and values he/she represents. Leaders are agents and catalysts through which others understand and identify with these ideas, purposes, and values, and are uplifted and motivated by them. When this occurs, a leader's efforts are amplified and focused in ways that enhance a company's competitive advantages and help it to serve society.
>
> (Badarocco and Ellsworth, 1989, p. 209)

I have known all three types of leaders. The political nurse leader will negotiate everything, which leads to organizational unrest. The directive leader seldom allows staff and first-line nurse managers to have input into decisions or freedom to be creative. The nurse leader who is values-driven is the one who will be most likely to encourage caring as the organizational goal. There are times when it is very hard to be a values-driven leader. There is always so much to do, and it seems so hard to be a catalyst. In the short term, it is easier to be directive, but that rarely results in employees that work with you to reach a goal such as caring. It seems like there are so many people who prefer to just leave things the way they are. This is a time when nurse leaders must not succumb to being directive.

They must strive to work with nurses in all kinds of roles to optimize the shared value of caring.

Hammer and Champy (1993) wrote a book about *Reengineering the Corporation* in which they say that many of today's corporations do not need little changes but complete reengineering. Rather than setting out to "fix things," the company must be willing to start all over again. This approach capitalizes on American values of individualism, self-reliance, willingness to accept risk, and propensity for change. The core message of the book is that it is no longer necessary or desirable for companies to organize their work like Adam Smith's bureaucratic division of labor. Now organizations must organize around process. Process is defined as a set of activities that, taken together, produce a result of value to a customer. Nurses operate using the nursing process. They understand that the real question we must ask about all the organizational activities is, "Are they what the customer wants or needs?" In nursing's case, the customer wants caring. These authors write that there are three forces driving today's companies: customers, competition, and change. The company must start over by abandoning long-established procedures and try to make them more responsive to the needs of customers, competition, and change. It is hard for nurses to abandon their ways. Hammer and Champy say that you seek breakthroughs, not by enhancing existing processes, but by discarding them and replacing them with entirely new ones that will create value to the customer. In this system, jobs will be redefined, which takes intelligence and responsibility. The authors call the new employees in these jobs "case workers." Interesting words when we consider that case management is becoming all the rage in health care. These authors say that the work gets done where it makes the most sense, and checks and controls are reduced. They talk about process teams that naturally fall together to complete a whole piece of work. Management roles change to providing resources, answering questions, and taking pride in the accomplishment of others. This book—like so many others we have reviewed—is calling for a new type of manager—one that values and works with all nurses toward a caring system. Again we are striving to have employees do work that is meaningful and managers who would rather be facilitators than bosses.

In nursing, there is not a lot written about leaders and organizations of the future. Porter-O'Grady (1986) wrote *Creative Nursing Administration:*

Participative Management into the 21st Century. As you may guess, this book is similar in many ways to the others we have reviewed. This nurse-author stresses that change is accelerating, and that participative strategies for the future are not optional but are absolutely necessary. He agrees with our other authors that managers must change traditional ways of managing. Managers and practitioners are closely interdependent. Managers must be able to share with professional colleagues more control and responsibility over the work itself. The role of the nurse manager becomes one of facilitating, coordinating, integrating, and supporting decisions, rather than one of controlling and directing. He describes participatory organizations as ones which:

1. value unity and coherence;

2. promote a sense of responsibility and awareness;

3. recognize interdependence and collaborative relationships;

4. make major decisions made at the practice level; and

5. understand the heavy demand for planning and involvement at all levels of the organization.

Benner and Wrubel (1989) reported the feelings of one staff nurse (Tracey White) who reported having a "love-hate" relationship with the profession of nursing: "We share this similar yet unarticulated frustration that there is much we are unable to do because of the bureaucracy of the hospital institution that dictates the volume of patients to be cared for by each nurse and increasingly forces us to accomplish the minimal and more obvious aspects of our care" (p. 365).

Benner and Wrubel point out that many nurses are suffering from "burnout," which can cause physical and emotional problems. "Besides respite and recreation, the person experiencing burnout needs to be reconnected to sustaining relationships and meanings to overcome the alienation and anomie" (p. 373). This type of burnout is often caused by expecting nurses to care and give care to too many patients. MacPherson (1989) says that part of the problem of having nurses in bureaucratic organizations is that their work is assumed to be quantifiable. For example, most patient classification systems do not account for the unquantifiable type of caring that we want nurses to practice.

Benner and Wrubel (1989) believe that a new vision of nurses as knowledge and caring workers is needed in organizations. Nurses need clinical promotion programs and participative management systems to increase their feelings of self-respect and organizational respect. These authors believe that nurses should sit on governing boards and central committees in order to shape their practices. "Empowering the practicing nurse is the best remedial action for organizational stress that nurses confront in hospital settings" (p. 388). They believe that nurses must be liberated to practice from a caring point of view, and organizations will have to be redesigned to facilitate this mission. By developing authentic caring relationships in work settings, nurses can experience satisfying feelings about their work. At the same time, the organization benefits by serving patients who feel cared for and thus can get well quicker. Through caring, patients often experience a special kind of love which assists them in their recovery or in providing an environment conducive for a peaceful death (Benner and Wrubel, 1989). Nursing administrators must see that the nurses feel loved as well.

So, what can we conclude form all this organizational literature? First, we learn that our world is moving too fast for the cumbersome bureaucracy to respond to all the changes in the organizational environment. Second, it is clear that the bureaucracy cannot meet the needs of today's employees. Third, we have learned that it is very hard to break away from the bureaucracy. We have seen that there are many new models of organizing—that current authors place great emphases on creativity, flexibility, and people-oriented organizations. There are new ways to manage—new ways to focus on organizational goals. It is amazing to me that so many authors have said the same thing over and over. It is encouraging and puzzling at the same time! Can so many authors be wrong or be ignored? Surely the business world cannot ignore all the emphasis on working better with employees and paying attention to their vision and goals. The question is, can we continue to move toward newer organizational models? Can the real world become more like the theoretical world?

This is an especially important question as we brace ourselves for major changes in the health care industry. We know that other industries who have been challenged have not reacted in a caring manner. But, health care is all about caring. As we are challenged economically, can we keep the caring in health care? The answer to that question will largely depend on nurses and, in particular, nurse administrators.

We have examined three types of management systems. In order to show their relationship to one another, the following schematic is proposed:

Organizational Theory

Bureaucratic Organizations (organizations as machines)	*Current Theoretic Organizations* (organizations as organisms)
1. Tight hierarchical structure	1. Loose structure
2. Workers as commodities	2. Valued employees
3. Strict rules for everything	3. Strong values, minimal rules
4. Depersonalized atmosphere	4. Individualized, open environment
5. Managers as bosses	5. Managers as facilitators
6. Standardized work	6. Flexible, variable work
7. Routine output	7. Variable output
8. Trained, consistent workers	8. Well-educated, independent employee

Caring Organizations

1. Loose structure, individual decision making
2. Colleagues of nurses at all levels—connectedness
3. Few rules—intimacy and values
4. Patient-centered atmosphere
5. Relationships as primary
6. Work is open to change and creativity
7. Individualized output
8. Skilled, knowledgeable professionals

In looking at the different management structures, it is plain that the caring organization resembles the current theoretical organizations much more than the bureaucracies, but I think even caring organizations need some structure provided by bureaucracies. Caring organizations are an extension of current organizational theories in that they encourage even more connectedness between people and more individuality in the finished product—patient care. Nurses must use all their knowledge and intuition to help patients find meaning and healing in their experience with the health care system.

In nursing, we have come a long way in "debureaucratizing" our nursing organizations. We have learned from books like Porter-O'Grady's (1986) *Creative Nursing Management* and the writings of countless nurse administrators who read the organizational books like those we have described. We have created organizational structures like participative management and shared governance and have seen the positive response of nurses who use their caring values and skills to create outstanding nursing departments. There are two problems, though, that I see on the horizon. First, not all nursing systems really use the caring process in structuring and operating their business. Second, many nurses and nurse administrators hang on tight to the familiar bureaucracy, and work continues to feel miserable in these organizations. Some nurse managers like the feeling of power that the bureaucracy provides, and some become so enmeshed in the overall hospital matters that they seem to leave behind all the lessons they learned about caring. Often it is not a conscious decision, but they forget to still be a nurse. No matter what the job, our nursing knowledge, and particularly the values of caring, must remain a central part of how we do our jobs. The intention of this book is to attempt to bring caring front and center for nurses and nurse administrators so that all of health care may benefit from the tradition of caring of which we are so proud. Certainly this literature can give us confidence to plunge ahead with creating caring nursing organizations.

References

Aldridge, Howard E. (1979) *Organizations and Environments.* Englewood Cliffs, NJ: Prentice.

Badaracco, J. L. and R. R. Ellsworth, (1989). *Leadership and the Quest for Integrity.* New York: Harvard Business School Press.

Benner, P. and J. Wrubel, (1989). *The Primacy of Caring: Stress and Coping in Health and Illness.* Menlo Park, CA: Addison-Wesley.

Boulding, K. E. (1978). General systems theory—the skeleton of science. In J.M. Shafritz and P.H. Whitbeck, eds., *Classics of Organization Theory.* Oak Park, IL: Moore Publishing Company, pp. 121–130.

Gillem, T. R. (1988). Deming's 14 points and hospital quality: Responding to the consumer's demand for the best value health care. *Journal of Nursing Quality Assurance* 2 (3): 70–78.

Hammer, M. and J. Champy, (1993). *Reengineering the Corporation.* New York: Harper Business.

Jackson, J., C. P. Morgan, and J.G.P. Paolilla, (1986). *Organizational Theory.* Oak Park, IL: Prentice-Hall.

Kantor, R. (1983). *Change Masters.* New York: Simon and Schuster.

Kotter, J. P. (1990). *A Force for Change: How Leadership Differs from Management.* New York: The Free Press.

Kramer, M. and C. Schmalenberg (1988). Magnet Hospitals: Part one and part two. *The Journal of Nursing Administration.* 18 (1): 13–24, 18 (2): 11–19.

Lawton, B. B. (1993). The American roots of Deming and quality. In Eisenach and Hansen eds. *Readings in Renewing American Civilization.* New York: McGraw Hill.

Lodahl, T. M., and S.M. Mitchell (1980). Drift in the development of innovative organizations. In J. K. Kimberly and R.H. Miles. *The Organizational Life Cycle.* San Francisco: Jossey-Bass Publishers.

MacPherson, K. I., (1989) A new perspective on nursing and caring in a corporate context. *Advances In Nursing Science* 11 (4): 32–39.

Marriner-Tomey, A. (1988). *A Guide to Nursing Management.* St. Louis: C.V. Mosby.

Morgan, G. (1986). *Images of Organizations.* Beverly Hills, CA: Sage Publications.

———. (1993). *Imagination: The Art of Creative Management.* Newbury Park, CA: Sage Publications.

Naisbitt, J. (1982). *Megatrends.* New York: Warner Books.

Naisbitt, J. and P. Auburdene (1990). *Megatrends 2000: Ten New Directions for the 1990s.* New York: William Morrow and Company.

Peters, T.J. (1992) *Liberation Management: Necessary Disorganization for the Nanosecond of the Nineties.* New York: A.A. Knopf.

Peters, T. J. and R. H. Waterman (1982). *In Search of Excellence.* New York: Harper and Row.

Porter-O'Grady, T. (1986). *Creative Nursing Administration: Participative Management for the 21st Century.* Rockville, MD: Aspen Publications.

Senge, P. M. (1990). *The Fifth Discipline: The Art and Practice of the Learning Organization.* New York: Doubleday Currency.

Taylor, F. W. (1978). The principles of scientific management. In J. M. Shafritz and P. H. Whitbeck, eds. *Classics of Organization Theory.* Oak Park, IL: Moore Publishing Company. pp. 23–37.

Watson, J. (1990). Caring knowledge and informed moral passion. *Advances in Nursing Science.* 13 (1): 15–24.

———. (1985). *Human Science and Human Care.* Norwalk, CT: Appleton-Century-Crofts.

Weber, M. (1978). Bureaucracy. In J. M. Shafritz and P.H. Whitbeck, eds., *Classics of Organization Theory.* Oak Park, Ill.: Moore Publishing Company. pp. 9–23.

Woodward, J. (1978). Management and technology. In J. M. Shafritz and P.H. Whitbeck, eds., *Classics of Organization Theory.* Oak Park, IL, Moore Publishing Company, Inc. pp. 190–205.

Young, L. C. and A.N. Hayne (1988). *Nursing Administration: From Concepts to Practice.* Philadelphia: W.B. Saunders.

CHAPTER FIVE

Leadership Styles

We have discussed leadership to some extent in the chapter on organizational theory. But it is a topic of such importance, I feel we need to expand on it here.

Leadership is, to me, the essence of nursing administration. Kotter (1990) reminded us that managers create stability and leaders create movement. Being the chief nurse executive gives one some latitude in how the job is defined. When I was an associate director of nursing, I thought I would never advance to the chief nurse executive job because mine was so much more fun. It seemed to me that my boss was so hemmed in by the system that she did not have time to do the more creative, fun things that I did. I was assigned to a lot of project work at first, and those days may have been the best in my career. I worked first on patient classification/utilization review, then on to implementing a quality assurance program, and then on to implementing primary nursing. Everything was fresh and new, and I had so much energy that I hardly noticed when the projects overlapped and I worked too hard. Not everything we tried worked (our career ladder bombed), but there were several other master's-prepared nurses, and we formed a very productive team.

Meanwhile, it seemed like my boss went to an infinite number of meetings and did endless paperwork. She was a very caring person, and she knew the names of most nurses, along with their husbands and children. I tried to pattern myself after her interpersonal skills. But eventually my boss left, and I had to decide whether to apply for the job. I told one of my friends about my fears of getting gobbled up by paper work and meetings. She replied that she, too, had noticed that about executives, but she believed that the executive had the authority to assign work any way he/she wanted. She suggested that some of the meetings and paper work could be delegated to leave room for creative, project-oriented work if I chose.

That sounded great to me, and it is just what I did. My first move was to put into place a small group of nurse administrators who could work with me as a team. I told them that I did not want the job if I had to do it by myself. They were enthusiastic. In the past, whenever a meeting came up that needed nursing representation, my boss would go. I divided the hospital into areas with nursing directors and I sent them to all the meetings involving their areas. Much of the paper work was reduced by letting other nurse managers sign them. We worked very hard to make the head nurses real good managers, and they took care of everything involving their units.

I still had more meetings and more paper work than I wanted, but I also had time for going to the units to interact with nurses and patients. And I continued to work on creative project development as well. It was a very important lesson for me to learn, and I just kind of stumbled on to it. So, my advise is that if you are interested in a new job or unhappy with the one you have, remember that you have the right and responsibility to create or re-create how your job is structured. The other piece of advice is to never stop learning.

There is a lot to learn about leadership. There have been hundreds of books written about the topic, so we will just touch on a few. Bennis and Nanus (1985) wrote that leadership is desired by almost everyone. But, once the enormity of present-day changes and challenges are realized, it does not feel so glamorous. Every author says we do not have enough good leaders. There is argument about whether leaders are born or taught. Kotter says that at least a part of being a leader is a fact of birth—those with higher IQs and assertive personalities are much more likely to lead. Everyone writes about what the new leader should be like. Bennis and

Nanus write about "transformative leadership" in which the leader is one who commits people to action, who converts followers into leaders, and may convert leaders into agents of change. These authors say that one out of four jobholders currently work at full potential, and six out of ten do not work as hard as they used to. Where leaders have failed, then, is to instill vision, meaning, and trust in their followers—to empower them to a higher level of performance. What is missing in today's businesses is "power, the basic energy to initiate and sustain action translating intention into reality" (p. 15). As we view it, effective leadership can move organizations from current to future states, create visions of potential opportunities for organizations, instill within employees commitment to change, and instill new cultures and strategies in organizations that mobilize and focus energy and resources" (p. 17).

These authors believe that problems will not be solved without effective leaders. Like Kotter, Bennis and Nanus see management and leadership as different. Bennis and Nanus see management's function as "to bring about; to accomplish; to have charge of or responsibility for, to conduct" (p. 21). Leading, however is "influencing, guiding in direction, course, action, and opinion" (p. 21). The distinction is crucial. Managers are people who do things right and leaders are people who do the right thing. I think, to some extent, that what I was struggling with in my job decision was that I wanted to be a leader, not a manager. I enjoyed the leadership parts of my job, and actually worried that those management skills were not what I did well. In my case, it was important for me to set up my job so I could lead, and hire others around me that might be better managers. Bennis and Nanus define four types of human skills that leaders must posses:

1. "Attention through vision"—results-oriented, compelling, clarity, concentration.

2. "Meaning through communication"—relate a compelling image, shared meanings, problem solving.

3. "Trust through positioning"—accountability, predictability, reliability, tireless persistence, and relentless dedication.

4. "Positive self-regard"—the higher the rank, the more interpersonal and human the undertaking—leaders trust the creative deployment of self.

Covey (1990) wrote *Principle-Centered Leadership,* in which he says that the highest level of human motivation is a sense of personal contribution. Principle-centered leadership focuses on work with fairness, kindness, efficiency, and effectiveness. People are not treated as just resources or assets, but also as spiritual beings who want meaning, a sense of doing something that matters. Where old leaders acted like cops, referees, devil's advocates, or naysayers, the new leader needs to act like a cheerleader, coach, facilitator, nurturer, and champion. The three basic categories on influence are to model by example ("others see"), to build caring relationships ("others feel"), and to mentor by instruction ("others hear").

Covey suggests seven habits of ineffective people:

1. Be reactive; doubt yourself, and blame others.
2. Work without any clear end in mind.
3. Do the urgent thing first.
4. Think win-lose.
5. Seek first to be understood.
6. If you can't win, compromise.
7. Fear change and put off improvement.

(Covey, 1990, p. 14)

Covey writes about principle-centered leadership as introducing a new paradigm that is influenced by laws of the universe such as fairness, equity, survival, and stability. He says that people instinctively trust those whose personality is founded on correct principles. Trust is key in the principle-oriented organization, and communication is easy, effortless, and instant. One of the characteristics of authentic leaders is their humility. Covey defined eight discernible characteristics of people who are principle-centered leaders:

1. "They are continually learning."

2. "They are service-oriented—see life as a mission."

3. "They radiate positive energy."

4. "They believe in other people—seek to believe in the unseen potential."

5. "They lead balanced lives—are not extremists. They see things as continuums, priorities, hierarchies. They courageously condemn the bad and champion the good."

6. "They see life as an adventure—savor life; their security lies in their initiative, resourcefulness, creativity, willpower, courage, stamina, and native intelligence. They rediscover people each time they meet them."

7. "They are synergistic ("synergy" is when the whole is more than the sum of its parts). They are change catalysts who work smart and hard to find new creative ways."

8. "They exercise for self-renewal—physical, mental, emotional, and spiritual." p. 39

Covey writes a lot about total-quality management, which he sees as the key to American success and survival. He says that total-quality management is the century's most profound, comprehensive alteration in management theory and practice. To achieve total-quality management, managers must become leaders, drawing from their people their greatest capacity to contribute ideas, creativity, innovative thinking, attention to detail, and analysis of process and product to the workplace.

Covey's ideas are congruent with the caring theory. His emphasis on managers being people-centered and employees as precious instead of throwaway commodities is exactly how I see caring management. I also believe in basing management on principles or values (depending on the author's key word), and I think the job ahead for managers is extremely chaotic. If managers do not have an anchor in principles, I think they have a tough road ahead. As Covey says, "We may have the right rhetoric, style, and intention, but without trust we may not achieve primary greatness or lasting success" (p. 58).

I know many managers who can spout out the latest management theory, but they do not get the message down deep, where it can change their practice. In nursing, I think we have a better chance to catch on to the new, more people-oriented theories because our work is so authentic. When dealing with people who are ill, you can't fake caring. The key for nurses who go into management is to carry authentic values with them and spread them around whenever possible. I knew one manager in particular (not in nursing) who was so very good at talking the values of quality management and people-oriented management. The problem was, he was a fake. He talked a good line when it was to his advantage, but if no one special was around, he was combative, demeaning, and anything but patient-centered. When the gloves came off, it was clear that his agenda was himself and hurting the people around him. I do not know if, when he reads books like Covey's, he really thinks he believes in it, but I do know that he lacks the basics—he is anything but a principle-centered manager. These kind of managers are everywhere you go. The problem becomes "How do I deal with them?" The only answer is for *you* to be the principle-centered manager who does not cave in to such pressures that can be applied. Just do not lose your authentic self and do your job the best way you can within the constraints of the situation.

Another author who writes like Covey is Barker (1992). He wrote that there are three keys for the future of any organization: 1. anticipation; 2. innovation; and 3. excellence. He says that the future is where our greatest leverage is and that you can and should shape your own future, because if you don't, someone else will. He says that, in the times ahead, good businesses must have the ability to look ahead—to anticipate. The ability to anticipate is enhanced by understanding what influences yourself, by divergent thinking and convergent thinking, by drawing pathways to the future, and by imaging in pictures or words or drawings what you see for the future.

Barker wrote a lot about paradigms, which he says are models, patterns, examples—the basic way you perceive the world. Paradigms are sets of rules and regulations that establishes boundaries and tell you how to behave in order to be successful. Organizations have many paradigms— management paradigms, sales paradigms, recruitment paradigms, and research and development paradigms. The problem with paradigms is that they change. For example, before Christopher Columbus sailed to the new world, everyone operated under the paradigm that the world was flat. A major paradigm had to change. It did not happen overnight. Some people continued to believe the old paradigm for a long time. Paradigms organize what we know and how we behave. They continue to be used until problems arise that cannot be solved by the paradigm, and then people have to look at other ways of behaving or believing. Barker says, "Every paradigm will, in the process of finding new problems, uncover problems it cannot solve. And these unsolvable problems provide the catalyst for triggering the paradigm shift" (p. 52).

Who changes the paradigm? Often it is a young person fresh out of school who has not totally bought into the paradigm. Or, it could be an older person who is shifting fields. Often it is the maverick in the organization, who is always questioning things as they are. Sometimes the paradigm will be challenged by the person who has run into a problem that cannot be solved, and he will not let go of the problem until he finds another kind of solution—one that may rock the foundations of a business or the world. Barker says the paradigm pioneer brings brains, brawn, time, effort, capital, and a lot of intuitive judgment. Those who choose to change their paradigms early, do it not as an act of the head but as an act of the heart.

Paradigms are changing all around us in today's world. As all these authors are trying to say, it is time to stop running organizations like the bureaucracy—the old paradigm—and build new organizations based on new values of flexibility, change, and people-orientedness. Health care is undergoing huge paradigm shifts. Things we thought impossible a few years ago are commonplace. And, the business of health care is undergoing a huge paradigm shift. Nursing is undergoing a paradigm shift as we see ourselves in more autonomous ways and try new treatments (which would have been unthinkable a few years ago). I see caring as a great and important paradigm shift that will open up new realities in nursing, in health care, and in the world. And we can be paradigm pioneers as we learn to apply the paradigm of caring. The caring paradigm is going great guns in the clinical setting of a few pioneers, and I believe it will move quickly into mainstream health care. I am not quite so optimistic about the implementation of the caring paradigm in health care management. The cost-reduction proposals rely on businesses that have nothing invested in health care except the bottom line. We have also discussed the difficulties of implementing caring in nursing management. So, the success of our caring paradigm will ultimately rest on the shoulders of nursing administrators. That is what this book is all about. It is about finding and knowing the caring paradigm, and then it is about how to make the caring paradigm come alive for nursing.

Nurses have abilities that can be very helpful in management. Agor (1984) wrote about intuitive management, which describes left-brained, right-brained, and integrated-brain management. Left-brained managers have traditionally received the most attention. They stress analytic and quantitative techniques and solve problems by breaking them down into manageable parts, then approaching the problem sequentially, relying on logic and data as tools in the process. Right-brained managers, however, rely primarily on feelings before facts when making decisions. Problems are solved by first looking at the whole, and often without total information or data at hand.

They reach decisions through intuitive insights or flashes of awareness that are received in four ways: 1. physically (bodily sensations); 2. mentally (mentally see pattern or order to seemingly unrelated facts); 3. emotionally (instantaneous like or dislike); or 4. spiritually (to come in touch with a sense of linking to all of humanity). The integrated-brain manager deals with facts *and* feelings, and tends to make major decisions guided by intuition after scanning the available facts and receiving input from management resources/personnel who are left- and right-brained in approach.

Caring is an intuitive matter. It relies on feelings and solving problems in a way that has meaning. In nursing, one must be an integrated-brain manager, as you use left-brain science and right-brained caring to deal with patient care settings that appreciate patients as total human beings.

Agor says, as do so many of the organizational writings, that we are in new times that will be constantly changing, crisis-oriented, with major structural changes. Individuals aspiring to top-level management jobs will need to possess a greater degree of right-brained skills, including intuition than ever before. Agor tested 2,000 managers to see about their management styles and found that the top executives used the integrated-brain approach most commonly. He also found that women scored higher on the right-brain approach. The author believes that you can develop intuition by keeping records of intuitive experiences, sharing your experiences with others, and eliminating interference that disrupts a free-flowing atmosphere. Other ideas to enhance your intuitive abilities include hypnosis, meditation, guided imagery, dream analysis, and biofeedback. Agor suggests that offices include comfortable seating, soft colors, music, and interpersonal communication. Managers should solicit information and carefully consider its meaning. He suggests staying, in part, a child with creativity and intention.

Nurses have been using intuition in their practice for many years, and it should be helpful as they become managers. Intuition is closely aligned with caring, and, if fully developed, is a highly efficient way of knowing. It is fast and accurate and can provide answers to problems that cannot always be clearly defined. In patient care settings, even physicians have great respect for nurses' intuitions, and as managers, it will become more and more useful.

Lee Iacocca (1988), the former chairman of the Chrysler Corporation, was very concerned about the direction management is going in this country. He wrote from years of experience, and his first admonition was to remember that the staff supports the boss. Without the staff, there is no need for a boss. He suggests that the boss can set a tone by saying these magic words: "I don't know," followed by, "but I'll find out." This acknowledges that business is nothing more than a bunch of human relations. You have to start with good people, lay out the rules, communicate with your employees, and motivate them. "Once you've laid down the rules, you have to sit back and trust your people, even though you won't know for awhile if they'll come through on the battlefield" (p. 79). His advise to leaders is:

1. Hire the best.
2. Get your priorities straight and keep a hot list of what you're trying to do.
3. Say it in English and keep it short.
4. Never forget the line makes the money.
5. Lay out the size of the playing field.
6. Keep some mavericks around.
7. Stay in business during alterations.
8. Remember the fundamentals.

When all is said and done, be yourself, stay natural, and dammit, smile once in awhile.

(Iacocca 1988, pp. 86–89)

Iacocca's book is important because it was not written by a theorist; it was written by a real boss. He says things much more pragmatically, and they are easy to read. But, even though he is not as theoretical about it, he says what everyone else does—appreciate your employees.

One of the ways I think you show appreciation to employees is by expecting a lot of them (within reason, of course). In general and in nursing, I have found that people will live up to whatever you expect of them, and they will feel a great deal of pride in their success. As Bennis and Nanus said, "The first thing you naturally do is to teach the person to feel that the undertaking is manifestly important and nearly impossible" (1985, p. 30). To have that attitude in nursing leadership is merely to paint an accurate picture of most nurses' jobs. Their work is so important that lives depend on it, and it is nearly impossible under current economic conditions.

I do not think I ever really understood how important nurses' work was until I became a patient. Ever since then, I tell every group of nurses I speak to just how important their work really is. The patient feels so vulnerable and the nurse is the only one around that you can reach to for help. They are your lifeline.

Styles (1982) wrote that nursing needs to emphasize:

1. understanding the social significance of their work;

2. committing to the ultimacy of professional performance (always working to your ultimate ability); and

3. respecting collegiality and collectively (feeling that all levels of nurses must work together).

The leader's job is to instill the desire for these three qualities and to work alongside all nurses to achieve them. I do believe there are times when nurse administrators have to make unpopular decisions. But, if they have the proper relationship with the nurses, the nurses will trust the nurse administrator to do what is best within a situation. The fact is that sometimes the administrator knows more about an issue than do the nurses as a whole. The nursing administrator cannot have a total laissez-faire style of leadership, but should strive for maximum input from staff nurses whenever possible.

Adams (1990) agrees that, in general, nurse administrators should identify themselves as democratic leaders who practice participative decision making. But there are times when a more autocratic approach may be needed. These times might include: 1. when information needed to make the decision cannot be widely shared; 2. when decisions must be made immediately; or 3. when nurses are unwilling to participate in decision making.

Some nurses are less positive about nursing leadership. Marriner-Tomey (1988) defines leadership as the ability to lead, guide, direct, or show the way. She wrote that nurses lack leadership skills because nursing attracts people who rank lower in self-esteem and initiative and higher in submissiveness and need for structure. She continues by saying that autocratic nursing leaders do not foster leadership in others, and that nurses may find leadership less than rewarding because of the conflicts with patient care, a stifling atmosphere, and autocratic systems.

These remarks are not consistent with what I see in nursing leaders of today. I think that they may have been true ten to twenty years ago, but the nurse administrators I meet today are not generally autocratic and do not feel conflicted in their jobs. In the past nurses have been submissive, but I do not see submissiveness or low self-esteem in nursing graduates today.

Young and Hayne (1988) wrote about power in leadership, which they define as the ability and willingness to affect the behavior of others. They list the key elements of power as strength, energy, positivism, optimism, and enthusiasm. They suggest that one way to acquire power is to assume you have it and act accordingly. These nursing authors suggest acquiring power by creating a good first impression, being caring and considerate, using sexuality (including a good wardrobe and doing your nails), and by using verbal power tools (rational thinking).

I had a very hard time with these ideas for acquiring power. It offends me to hear such advise in this day and age. Obviously, anyone who does not know how to dress well may have a problem, but there are much more crucial issues for power in leadership. My impression of how nursing leaders acquire power is simple: be competent. Learn management theory, learn more about nursing theory, learn how the system works in your organization, and use all your skills covered with a layer of caring. I think that nurse leaders of today show their power using intuitive as well as rational thinking, and that they have gained the respect of their nurse colleagues and other administrators throughout the health care industry. I see nurse administrators with energy, and they are people that are getting promoted in the organizational hierarchy. We have power because we are knowledgeable, sensitive, competent leaders who can formulate long-term, society-based, caring business decisions.

Another nurse author (Murphy 1990) suggests that nurses are not necessarily good followers. She wrote of a description of followers as:

1. Sheep—incapable of critical thinking and lacking initiative and a sense of responsibility.

2. Yes-people—often young nurses who are not enterprising, giving way to the opinions and decisions of others.

3. Alienated—capable of critical thinking and independence, but often using their capabilities to resist and oppose leaders. They often see themselves as always right, better than any boss.

4. Survivor—plays things safe, work for service pins and act like melting jello.

5. Effective follower—think for themselves, have initiative, have commitment beyond themselves.

Murphy lists strategies for developing effective followers as: 1. recognize their value; 2. offering nurse follower training at orientation; and 3. making the roles of followers and leaders more equally important to success.

As you might guess, I did not like Murphy's description of followership. I will bet you won't have a crowd in her class on followers. I think there is value to addressing followership as a concept, but if we do, four of the five categories should not be negative and demeaning. I think we need to see all roles as partially following and partially leading. A staff nurse leads in patient care and follows in relation to her boss. The chief nurse executive leads in nursing but is a follower to the board of directors. In this book, we have talked some about how the followers should sometimes lead. Instead of trying to figure out who is following and leading, we need to put our energy into positive experiences of working together without reference to rank. We, especially in nursing, need to work together in a caring way as colleagues. Occasionally, I have heard leaders say disparaging things about staff nurses; more often, I have heard staff nurses say things like, "You're not a real nurse, what do you know about nurses in the trenches?" Instead of fussing about our differences, why can't we understand that every nurse is performing a key role, whether they are staff, middle managers, or top administrators?

Some of the bad feelings about leaders are indeed justified. Kantor (1983) writes that rarely in tradition-bound organizations do bosses actually have to say no to subordinates. They do it with a well-placed frown, a raised eyebrow, or pregnant pauses. Most people in organizations never bother to pursue new ideas, because of the "failure of success." It is rare to find a boss who actually encourages innovation by rewarding successful ideas and not punishing for the ones that do not work. Employees have to feel free of risk and rewarded for coming up with new ideas in the company.

Kantor suggests that success breeds success. If supervisors have high expectations, nurses can reach them with encouragement. People in the organization must be made to feel important, and if so, they can produce all kinds of improvements and new ideas. Kantor says to look to people inside the organization for ideas instead of hiring from outside the organization. She says we need to breed "cultures of pride" by developing a willingness to work together to find new ways of doing things. Kantor's climates of success and pride include:

1. Emotional and value commitment between person and organization.
2. People feel they "belong" to a meaningful entity. They can realize cherished values by their contributions; they have a sense of uniqueness and jointness.
3. Culture—encourages a tradition of change. Opinion leaders are innovative if the organization normally favors change.
4. Pride in the company. Innovation is the mainstream.
5. Feeling that people inside the company are competent leaders—don't rely on outsiders—invest heavily in management training.
6. High degree of organizational esteem.
7. Culture of pride based on high performance.
8. Mutual respect makes teamwork easier.
9. Supervisors hold high expectations of subordinates.
10. Formal awards and public recognition.
11. Performance stimulating pride stimulating performance.
12. People-centered focus.
13. Concerned with honesty and fairness.
14. Rewards—emphasizes investment in people and projects rather than payment for past service.

(Kantor 1983, pp. 142–154)

Kantor's ideas are very applicable to nursing. So many nursing environments are stifling and closed to new ideas. "This is the way we've always done it" is heard over and over. Our systems are so complex and leaders are so harried to get the management tasks done that there is no one listening for ideas. Then if one pops out, there are several layers of the hierarchy that can give that frown or raised eyebrow. Everywhere I go to speak to nurses, I ask for ideas for saving money, and I always get many very good ideas. But when I encourage them to tell someone about their ideas, they cannot think of anyone who will listen, let alone do something about it. Maybe we need an idea officer or a contest to see which team can come up with a new idea, and then we must give them a reward commensurate with the idea.

Laschinger and Havens (1996) did a study that supported Kantor's view that work structures have an impact on factors that influence employees' work effectiveness. In particular, control over professional nursing practice enhances work satisfaction. Organizations must include structures that allow empowered staff members to best manage their work within highly effective teams. In Laschinger and Havens' study, nurses felt moderately empowered with a moderate degree of control over their practice. There was a strong positive correlation between access to empowerment structures and their overall work satisfaction. This is an example of how caring is important to nurses and their organizations. A nurse needs to have control over work structures so that they may incorporate caring into their work, and satisfaction equals caring to a great extent in nursing.

During her experience as a patient, Belanger (1996) perceived the health care system to be focused on technical treatments and the bottom line, rather than on healing. She felt dissatisfaction and fear from staff, who seemed to be suppressed, angry, distrustful, wounded, and tense. Belanger feels that current health care initiatives such as work redesign, continuous improvement, reengineering, downsizing, and mergers are not going to heal the heart and soul of health care. Nurses are expected to leave themselves at home and be "professional." Belanger feels that the split between work life and our soul life at is the root of much of nursing's unhappiness. She advocates for organizations to create "healing environments" where we recognize that patients and nurses bring heart and soul to their situations. Everyone in the organization has to be willing to help create a healing environment that is joyous, peaceful, and whole. Leaders must speak the truth, accept truth from others, master the amount of feedback, own their contribution to problems, be willing to ask for help, be clear about what they want, and be themselves.

Nurse managers have a large impact on nurses' work and satisfaction. Edwards and Roemer (1996) wrote about nurse managers as key to the operation and adaptation of health care organizations because they manage large quantities of human, financial, and technological resources. Nurse managers should focus on external and internal environments to identify knowledge and skills necessary to be effective managers. "Nurse managers should be selected for their ability to manage all facets of the larger organization and community" (p. 13). Although nurse managers' skills must focus on identifying needs inside and outside the organization, they must maintain nurses' goals, which focus on patient care. If managers believe that caring is an important facet in organizational effectiveness, this value will be communicated to staff nurses who can take the managers' lead to make caring an important goal.

In the last few years there have been many organizational changes, and nurses have often gotten promotions. I am all for that! But Singleton and Nail (1988) urge us to give some thought to what that means for nursing. Many nurse executives are now vice president of patient care services, and they are performing very well. The biggest advantage is that it gives the nurse administrator the opportunity to coordinate patient care by being in charge of departments other than nursing. But Singleton and Nail ask the question, "What happens to the nursing organization when the structure is decentralized and no one fills the function of the traditional DON?" (p. 11). The new vice president of patient services must pay equal attention to several departments, and by sheer size nursing may need more direction than she can now afford to give. Wolf (1990) calls it "executive seduction." In their efforts to be equal to other departments, one may forget that the nurse executive has always been the leader of a professional discipline. Being leading nursing is not the same as managing regular employees. If this book is about anything, it is about growing professionally through a caring strategy. It is important to ask "who leads this difficult transition?" I believe it is an important issue for all vice presidents of patient care services. As McCloskey (1991) said: "The job of the nurse administrator is to create and maintain an environment within which professional nursing can be practiced. A good environment does not just happen—leadership is required to bring it about" (p. 5). Whether the vice president of patient care services chooses to hire a new director of nursing or tend to nursing herself, it is imperative that the professional development of nursing does not stop going forward. On the other side of the administrator's role, the vice president should use his/her influence to see that the whole organization is patient-centered. This organizational norm is crucial to optimal nursing practice.

McClosky also reminds us that not everything in administration has to be all serious. She advocates that nurse administrators approach their jobs as "Creating an Environment for Success with Fun, Hope, and Trouble" (p. 5). She thinks that if a job is fun to do, it is more satisfying and performance improves. She advocates having "big fun and little fun." Little fun involves amusement and joking and may include parties and such. Big fun is "the good feeling we get from being creative, making others feel good and being good at what we do" (p. 6). Another ingredient in maintaining a productive environment is hope. Hope is strength-giving, and involves believing that we can do things that matter. The last ingredient is trouble. It's what we get when we challenge the system. But to accomplish big dreams, it requires some risk taking and conflict. The trouble we speak of is not mean and unpleasant and creating roadblocks for the system. But we desperately need those mavericks who insist we look at things in a new way. They are the yeast that makes the bread of the system rise to new heights of performance. Trouble is a necessary part of excellence.

Most leaders are taught to focus on interpersonal relationships (the way leaders behave with other people). They fail to connect the intrapersonal (what one thinks within themselves) domain of the leader with the interpersonal relationships of the environment (Farrell and Nuttal, 1997). In other words, most leaders are more interested in how they can gain personally from their leading rather than how they can help others with their leadership. These authors have developed a way to help leaders identify their deeply held beliefs and the way they affect their leadership behavior. Farrell and Nuttal use face-to-face interviews, questionnaires, and self and organizational assessment instruments. This method ensured that the leaders went beyond superficial values to identify their deeper values and goals. These values affect the way these leaders make decisions and treat people. The authors meet with the leaders for four to six hours for feedback about their deeply held beliefs and values in their everyday work. Farrell and Nuttal wrote, "Our research with leaders has indicated to us that, given the opportunity, a deeper inter-human connectiveness, such as caring, exists" (p. 42).

I have always been frustrated by the fact that people can be taught new and caring leadership theories and yet many of them will not integrate the new knowledge into their work relationships. The Farrell and Nuttal method of identifying deep values and then helping leaders to consciously use these values in their work sounds like a very expensive but also very effective method for increasing understanding and application of, for example, caring values in the work setting. Caring is more than a belief; it needs to be lived by many leaders in an organization to create a caring organization.

A new term in management is "transformational management." Curtin (1997) wrote about transactional and transformational leaders. Transactional leaders approach followers with an eye to exchanging one thing for another. The employees know the leader is manipulating them and will support the leader only if it meets their own goals. This reminds me of the political leader described by Badaracco and Ellsworth.

Curtin describes the transformational leader as one who depends on mutual self-interests and taps into ideals that transcend self-interest to stimulate people and their organizations. Transformational leaders convert followers into leaders who are motivated by something more than self-interest. This is particularly important in health care because the people are administering care to people who are vulnerable and have critical human needs. Since transformational leadership involves worthy goals, Curtin is mystified by health care leaders who appeal to saving money or reducing costs as reasons for transforming their organizations. Why ask people to save money unless the savings will be used for worthy causes such as improved patient care?

I have a big dilemma when I think of leadership styles and the way organizations really are. My guess is that if you asked a hundred nurse leaders what their leadership style is, 95 percent would say "democratic" or "participative" or some such term. But when I talk to nurses, that is not at all the picture they display. A report in the *Journal of Nursing Administration* (Jolma, 1990) reported that, despite the recent trend toward decentralizing nursing management, nurses responding to a survey indicated a low perceived level of participation in decision making. I think staff nurses would say that 10 or 20 percent of nurse leaders are democratic or participative. I certainly thought I was participatory, but was I really? And, how can you find that out about yourself? I do believe that styles of leadership can change as people try to become less autocratic. But I still think there is a wide disparity between our own perceptions and those of people who work with us.

One exercise I have used to try to get leaders to understand themselves is the Keirsey and Bates (1978) exercise from their book *Please Understand Me*. The premise of the book is that people are different from one another, but that is not necessarily good or bad. And unfortunately we see other's differences as flaws and strive to change them to be like us. We want to sculpt people to be just like us, yet that fails before it begins. These authors advocate getting to know your own self and others and then using the differences in positive ways. They have a test you can take to type your personality. It measures introversion and extroversion, and it measures whether one sees the world from their senses (sight, smell, etc.) or from a more intuitive way. It also measures whether you are a person who wants closure to things or if you prefer to keep things open-ended. After you take the test, there are four personality types, according to the authors. Keirsey and Bates then describe the four types, and explain in detail why some types will be compatible at work and others will be at war.

When I first became the chief nurse executive, we hired a facilitator who used this test. We gathered all kinds of nursing leaders (head nurses, supervisors, quality assurance nurses, assistant directors of nursing, infection control nurses, discharge planning nurses). After a couple of hours of warm-up exercises and talk from the facilitator, we took the test. Then he asked us to move to a part of the room designated for people of our personality types. Strangely enough, there were only four (out of forty) people in my group. As the facilitator began to describe our group, he told us that it was an unusual type and why. He began to describe people of that personality type and how they tend to work, and one of the assistant directors of nursing jumped up and hollered to me, "That's why I can't understand how you do things!" It was a light-hearted, positive meeting, but we all came away a little bit wiser about ourselves and our colleagues. It was really very helpful to look at people's types and try to be understanding of their actions. I learned a lot about myself: that I was only slightly extroverted and that I think intuitively and want to keep things open and flowing. Now I could understand if someone told me I was indecisive when my main aim as a leader was to keep processes going. I took the test again a couple of years ago, and I found that my personality type had changed slightly. I do not know if that is good or bad.

But, for all nurse leaders, I highly recommend that you find experiences that bring you to understand yourself and then find ways to help others to understand you. One time when I was teaching nursing administration, we videotaped the students giving short presentations. People were shocked at what they saw. One person blurted out, "That's not anything like me!" and the class said, "Oh yes it is!" So outside feedback can be very helpful. I also believe strongly in introspection. We can look back each day or week and ask ourselves, "Was this an autocratic, democratic,

A Caring Approach in Nursing Administration

or participative, or laissez-faire decision? What was the most appropriate style for the occasion, and did I handle it in a caring way?" If you are lucky, as I have been, you may have a couple of very close colleagues who are brave enough to give you honest feedback. And just keep working for the goal—to be a caring nurse manager!

References

Adams, C. (1990). Leadership behavior of CNEs. *Nursing Management* (August): 36–39.

Agor, W. H. (1984). *Intuitive Management: Integrating Left and Right Brain Management Skills: How to Make the Right Decision at the Right Time.* Englewood Cliffs, NJ: Prentice Hall.

Barker, J. A. (1992). *Future Edge.* New York: William Morrow and Co., Inc.

Belanger, R. W. (1996). Leadership in a healing environment. *Seminars for Nurse Managers* 4 (4): 218–225.

Bennis, W. and B. Nanus (1985). *Leaders: Strategies for Taking Charge.* New York: Harper and Row.

Covey, S. R. (1990). *Principle-Centered Leadership.* New York: A Fireside Book by Simon and Schuster.

Curtin, L. (1997). How—and how not—to be a transformational leaders. *Nursing Management* 28 (5): 39–43.

Edwards, P. A. and L. Roemer (1996). Are nurse managers ready for current challenges of health care? *The Journal of Nursing Administration* 26 (9): 11–17.

Farrell, T. and G. Nuttal (1997). Influencing the caring capacity of leaders: The challenge of the work environment. *International Journal for Human Caring* 1 (1): 29–38.

Iacocca, L. (1988). *Talking Straight.* New York: Bantam Books.

Jolma, D. J. (1990). Participation, decision making, and job stress. *The Journal of Nursing Administration* 20 (9): 50.

Kantor, R. (1983). *Change Masters.* New York: Simon and Schuster.

Keirsey, D. and M. Bates (1978) *Please Understand Me.* Del Mar, CA: Prometheus Nemesis Books.

Kotter, J. P. (1990). *A Force for Change: How Leadership Differs from Management.* New York: The Free Press.

Laschinger, H.K.S. and D. S. Havens (1996). Staff nurse work empowerment and perceived control over nursing practice. *The Journal of Nursing Administration* 26 (9): 27–34.

McCloskey, J. C. (1991). Creating an environment for success with fun, hope, and trouble. *The Journal of Nursing Administration* 21 (4): 5–6.

Marriner-Tomey, A. (1988). *Guide to Nursing Management.* St. Louis: C. V. Mosby.

Murphy, D. (1990). Followers for a new era. *Nursing Management* 2 (7): 68–69.

Singleton, E. K. and F. C. Nail (1988). Nursing leadership: the effects of organizational structure. *The Journal of Nursing Administration* 18 (10): 10–14.

Styles, M. M. (1982). *On Nursing: Toward a New Endowment.* St. Louis: C. V. Mosby.

Wolf, G. (1990). Executive seduction. *The Journal of Nursing Administration* 20 (7/8): 10–11.

Young, F. W. and A. N. Hayne (1988). *Nursing Administration: From Concepts to Practice.* Philadelphia: W. B. Saunders.

CHAPTER SIX

The Health Care System

The purpose of this chapter is to examine the health care industry to see if it is, or can be, a caring system. We will not be examining individual care, which is most often very caring. We will be interested in the question, "Is the American health care system caring in nature?" It depends on where you are in the system when you judge the caring quality of the system. In the past, health care was seen as something that was viewed with compassion. You would hear, "If you have your health, you have everything." If someone got sick, everyone helped in whatever way they could. That is often still true on an individual basis, but I believe that the health care *system* has changed in character. There is no longer a sense of health care as a compassionate business.

You will recall from chapter two that Ray (1989) did a survey that indicated that everyone in the hospital felt that the work they did was caring. I suppose that is true of the whole industry, but sometimes it is very hard to see. I know a patient that is having problems with her jaw due to an auto accident. The insurance company, in its infinite wisdom, has refused to pay for physical therapy, which would probably correct the problem. Because of the "uncaring" insurance company, the patient will probably have to have surgery to correct the problem. Yet, yesterday I spoke to a nurse that works for an insurance company, and she insists that, in her job as a reviewer, her first priority is to obtain necessary caring services for her patients. Perhaps part of the problem lies in who defines caring services. Nurses will tell you that they believe that their actions for patients are indeed caring, but they do not believe that the whole system is caring. In fact, they will tell you that they must spend a great deal of energy working around the system in order to care properly for patients. The nurses feel that the increasingly money-hungry, business part of health care is making it harder and harder to be caring to patients.

What has caused health care to become more of a business and less of a compassionate industry? Part of the reason is that all of American businesses have taken on a much more money-oriented approach, and, as health care has taken up more and more of our nation's wealth, people have become less tolerant about costs. Most people do not understand why health care costs have increased so fast. They are unaware of the increased costs that come with each new piece of equipment, yet they want our health care system to find more and more ways to save lives and reduce suffering. They do not see that the health care system is delivering a much different product now than it was ten years ago. They just know that it costs a whole lot more. This chapter will explore some of the changes in product and attitudes concerning health care. It will be an unsettling chapter, because the pressures are creating an uneasy and frustrating atmosphere for health care professionals. We are used to being the "good guys" who make people feel better. It is difficult to be seen as a problem industry in our country. We must look at the problem of the health care system, though, so that we can determine what actions might make things more caring in our eyes and in the eyes of the people we serve. For, if we cannot find answers, our frustration at trying to be caring will grow.

While health care becomes more businesslike, Reinhardt (1986) challenged the assumption that America has the best health care system in the world. He points out that many people in the United States have no health care at all, because middle- and upper-income Americans are increasingly reluctant to purchase health care for low-income families. Reinhardt wrote that much of our frustration about health care comes from our inability as a nation to define ethically whether health care should be a basic right or a private consumer good that should be financed by individual recipients. The issue is that no one wants to pay for health care for all, yet no one wants to pay for all of their own health care. Fuchs (1988) believes that the 1980s witnessed a reversal of the egalitarian ethics of the 1960s and 1970s, when the national goal was to provide high-quality health care for all Americans. He wrote that the move toward competitiveness in the health care industry had little effect on overall expenditures. It has, however, had a big impact on the values of health care; it has indeed diminished caring in the health care system.

Reinhardt also draws attention to the fact that America has developed a health care financing system that has absurd parts. Our insurance system is fragmented and extremely expensive to administer. Our cost-containment measures so far have resulted in more administrators and more-complex financial systems. The effect on health care itself has been to reduce caring and to reduce services to many people. Reinhardt also wrote that part of the reason we ignore the plight of the poor is that Americans take a hard-nosed approach toward the poor. We seem to believe that poverty tends to be self-inflicted. In European democracies, poverty is viewed more as misfortune that is beyond the control of the individual. In addition, Americans are so suspicious of "big government" that they are more willing to ignore the poor than they are to establish tax-financed entitlements.

Reinhardt (1994) says that the providers of health care seek to give their patients the maximum feasible degree of physical relief, but overall they also seek a large slice of the gross national product as reward for their efforts. Patients also seek the maximum feasible degree of physical relief, but collectively they want to minimize the amount of the gross national product that must be spent on the health care system. Reinhardt also notes that most countries that have national health care systems limit the supply side of medical care—they limit the numbers of hospitals or doctors in their system, limit big-ticket technology, impose stiff price and budgetary controls, and limit overall expenditures. In the United States, we have let the supply side of health care control itself, and thus we have too many hospitals and doctors. We are trying to control the system now by demand factors such as utilization review systems and rationing care (a very new and controversial practice). Rationing is when someone decides that you cannot have health care even if you need it. Some kind of board or commission regulates who gets what. We have rationing now in that many Americans have no access to health care. Some states (Oregon was the first) are more explicitly rationing by refusing to pay for certain procedures for Medicaid patients.

Richard Lamm, the former governor of Colorado, has been an outspoken advocate for health care rationing for many years. He says that everybody recognizes the need to contain health care costs, but at the same time, Americans believe that everyone is entitled to unlimited health care, regardless of the cost. If current trends continue, our entire gross national product could be spent on health care in about seventy years. At this point, high health care costs have a huge impact on our economy. For example, $700 of the cost of each new car is spent on health care costs for the carmaker's employees. Lamm feels that unless we give more thought to how to prioritize our limited health care costs, we shall be bankrupt as a country.

One way to tell how caring the systems are is to look at some numbers. In 1990 there were 7 million health care workers (Feeney 1994). Lee and Estes (1994) wrote that Americans expended $800 billion on health care, a total of 14 percent of our gross national product (GNP). Yet the life expectancy for men ranked twentieth in the industrialized world, and women's life expectancy was fifteenth in the world (Rice, 1994). The use of medical services had an inverse relationship with income. Infant mortality remains high, cancer deaths continue to rise, and accidents are the leading cause of deaths among children and youth. Illicit drug use continues to be a problem, and the incidence, prevalence, and deaths from AIDS continue to rise. In 1960, the cost for health care to households was $143 per year; by 1988, it had risen to $2,124 per year. From 1960 to 1988, the growth in the GNP was 9.5 times; in health care the costs rose twenty times.

The frail elderly are the group that presents the greatest challenge. Those over eighty-five are now the fastest-growing population. In 1900, 4 percent of the population were elderly: in 1980 they were 11.3 percent, and by the year 2000, it is expected that one in every five Americans will be sixty-five and over. Even though the elderly are now about 12 percent of the population, they use up 36 percent of the health expenditures.

In 1990, the spending for health care in the United States exceeded Canada by 41 percent, France by 85 percent, Germany by 87 percent, Japan by 131 percent, Italy by 152 percent, and England by 171 percent. And yet all these countries have access to health care for all their citizens.

In the United States, there are about 37 million uninsured—15.5 percent of the population. Of these people, one-half are employed (75 percent if you include dependents). In addition, many more people are underinsured. As businesses try to solve their soaring health care costs, they have passed on much more of the costs to the individual worker through higher deductibles and copayments. Rice wrote that

> it is time for the federal government to assume responsibility in providing health care to its citizens. . . . it is not difficult to conclude that the vast expenditures for medical care in this country are providing neither universal access nor the highest health status that many other developed countries enjoy for a proportionately smaller expenditure. Nor is it difficult to conclude that providing universal and affordable health care is the major health priority, requiring a commitment by the people of the U.S. and its leaders.
> (Rice 1994, pp. 57–58)

There are many health care policy people who echo Rice's sentiment. Lee and Estes (1994) wrote that our nation is confronted by an outmoded system that is the result of failed policies and runaway technological expansion at the expense of the provision of sound basic care for all.

It is interesting to me that people are so frightened about health care reform. They say we cannot afford it, yet is has been documented that the cost of care for the currently uninsured is high because they cannot afford to get health care for routine things, which turn into major things, which cost much more to treat than if they were handled earlier. People say that the government would be more bureaucratic and clumsy than our current system. One has only to suffer a major illness to understand that the current system is impossible to deal with. There are over 1,300 insurance companies, and each has different forms and coverage parameters. Physicians are extremely burdened with paperwork, and patients are overwhelmed with trying to understand the whole health care system. The public says that a government system would become a mess like Medicare, but the truth about Medicare is that it is effectively run for many people. The biggest complaint about Medicare and Medicaid is that they reimburse low, and so patients need supplemental policies to cover all their health care costs. Critics of a government system say we would have long waits to see doctors or have surgeries, but I do not think people stop to think that we already spend so much more on health care than other nations, and that we would not necessarily have to limit our system to the extent that other countries do. The basic fact of the health care system is that it cannot be categorized as caring when it discriminates against so many.

Torrens and Williams (1994) describe our health care system as a circular gaming system. The rapid rise of the health care costs sets off a series of events that ultimately affect the entire American economy. The employers and insurance programs are forced to take cost-containment efforts that impact the providers to find more sources of revenue, which in turn affect the patients and communities. The circular system encourages each part of the system to figure out how to play the game.

In my city, for example, every hospital is scrambling to get costs down. Cuts in personnel (including nurses) are common, and hospitals and other health care organizations are banding together to become huge conglomerates. Health care organizations are willing to give up their autonomy because they are so frightened that independent organizations can no longer survive. This movement into conglomerates results in economies of scale and increased power for the larger systems. Health care workers are frightened about job security and losing the organizational camaraderie of smaller institutions. We have yet to learn just what this consolidation phase has in store for professionals or patients. In addition, many organizations are being bought by for-profit organizations where pressure for cost reduction is even greater. The mission of meeting community health needs becomes the goal of providing adequate care *and* making a profit.

Health care providers are also involved with creating their own health maintenance organizations (HMOs) and preferred physician organizations (PPOs) in the hope that they can capture patient markets. There is a move to integrate all health care services (out-patient surgeries and clinics, home care, hospice services, etc.) to be under the control of the conglomerate to maintain their patient base through all their health care needs. As yet, there is no evidence that these moves will reduce costs or maintain quality (although most conglomerates recognize that some amount of quality is necessary for business success).

All of this feels like a whirlwind of activities and change, and health care employees feel enormous pressure to cut costs. Yet an article came out in the paper a few weeks ago announcing that hospitals in our state had record profits last year. It must be very discouraging to a nurse who is being asked to care for more and sicker patients—to feel like she does not have time to be caring—to see that the results of her efforts was a healthy bottom line instead of happy, well-cared-for patients.

Torrens and Williams (1994) say that the reasons for cost increases could be seen as successes because: 1. we have more hospitals and hospital beds than we need; 2. we have more doctors than we need; and 3. we have had a remarkable growth in medical science and technology. The failure is our lack of willingness to develop a system that would integrate, supervise, and control these developments. We have all kinds of cost-control systems in place. The most aggressive are by health care insurance companies who are decreasing benefits, increasing deductibles and copayments, decreasing mental health benefits, and implementing rigorous utilization review. Actions taken by providers include downsizing hospitals, marketing, advertising, developing product lines, and working more closely with their doctors. Nurses and other therapists are developing new outpatient and home care services as independent businesses. The great irony, say Torrens and Williams, is that none of these have resulted in significant control of costs. Health care is bogged down in problems it did not create itself and cannot solve by itself. These authors think that every health care provider must understand that control of costs is his/her primary responsibility. While I believe that all providers have a responsibility to help bring costs down, I do not agree that it is their primary responsibility. Perhaps it is for the finance people, but the clinical people must always make patient welfare their top priority. It is frightening to see health policy experts leaving patients out of the equation.

This reminds us of what we learned about organizational and leadership theory. If organizations are to survive, they must be flexible, innovative, open, and respectful of employees. In the rush to survive in the marketplace, many health care organizations are listening only to the pressures of the environment, and are not focusing on employees and how health care professionals can change the system given the flexibility and autonomy to see new ways of doing things. Nurses can also be an innovative asset to health care organizations that want to focus on wellness instead of illness. I believe nursing can become a strong force in teaching patients about healthy lifestyles to reduce acute illnesses in our society, and that nurses will do so in a caring manner.

McKeown (1994) asks that we take a look at the determinants of health. We are so locked into the medical and business models that we forget that the biggest determinants of health have to do with pollutants and lifestyle. He says that medicine has taken an engineering approach to health care—assuming that the body is a machine that you can take apart and put back together. There is neglect of sick people whose ailments are not within the scope of the scientific theory. This author believes that the role of medicine in treating disease is overrated, and yet societies invest in health care rather than social programs that may, in the end, do more to keep people well.

Much blame for the excessive health care costs have been attributed to physicians. They were said to have no interest in containing costs, because it did not affect them personally until recently. Much has been made of defensive medicine, where physicians order more tests than necessary because they have been afraid of lawsuits. They did more than was necessary so that no one could say they did not do enough. As doctors' incomes rose quickly, they lost the trust of the public, who no longer thought that doctors were more interested in them than in the money they generated. As physicians became entangled with ownership of labs and joint ventures with hospitals, the public had further evidence that the doctor was no longer the simple, honest, competent vender of medical services, and the government and insurance companies began thinking of ways to control physicians' practices. In 1992, Congress passed a bill forbidding physicians from billing for labs in which the physician had an equity interest.

Now there are all sorts of regulations for physicians. Perhaps the most degrading is utilization review, where a nurse can decide to cut off a patient's benefits even when the doctor believes they are necessary. New efforts to develop "standards of care" or "practice protocols" has left many physicians feeling that medicine will soon be nothing but "cook-book medicine." Relman (1994) says that the old rewards of importance of service, personal responsibility without interference, the stimulation of science, and a secure livelihood are gone. Relman states that physicians should be competent, compassionate, and avoid ties with the health care market. Eddy (1994) says that the assumption that the physician's decision is always right is being challenged from many directions. Because of that challenge, we are creating elaborate systems to review the physician's

A Caring Approach in Nursing Administration

decisions. The problem is that we are using nurses and doctors who do not even *know* the patient to determine correctness, and how can we know if their decisions are any more correct? In one study, cases were deemed inappropriate in just 15 percent of cases, and physician appeals brought it down to 9 percent. However, Eddy believes physicians should not view these control mechanisms as a sinister plot, but as a sincere attempt to get a handle on costs and define what is quality care. The sad truth is that we lack the ability to compare different kinds of medical, social, and financial benefits. At some point we must come to grips with the fact that health care is not a pure science that can be precisely measured and controlled; much of health care is indeed a caring art.

Nursing is struggling mightily with the issue of equating patient outcomes to costs. It is very hard to sort out what effects are directly attributable to nursing, and our concepts of caring are the hardest of all to measure. As we must remember that part of medicine is an art that is difficult to measure, we also must conclude that a large part of nursing is an art. But rather than passively doing nothing about it, we must put our most creative energy to work on it. I am involved in a current demonstration project that measures patients' perceptions of nursing outcomes. The study is designed to measure caring outcomes, in particular after the nurses receive forty-six hours of education about caring and caring/healing treatments. We are trying to obtain the objective measures of caring required by today's health care evaluation systems.

Shore and Levinson obviously understand the art, as they wrote:

> The push is clearly on to make the delivery of health services more businesslike. . . . in the process of becoming successful businesses, hospitals and, by implication, health professionals as well may lose the quality of caring that has been one root of public trust and the most important aspect of personal and institutional identity in the health care field . . . An expedient preoccupation with the bottom line, productivity, and the efficient use of resources at the expense of human care and high professional standards will put the institution at a competitive disadvantage.
>
> (1986, p. 321)

Ten years after writing these words, I wonder how those authors feel. Certainly some of the predictions have come true—public trust in doctors and hospitals is at an all-time low, while preoccupation with the bottom line gets more and more intense. I do not believe at this time that nurses have become caught up in that mistrust, but we may be if we do not really focus on implementing caring—for patients and for the health care system.

I know that some nurses work solely for the business end of health care today, but you can work the business side with an eye on patient care. The fact is, we need nurses to work the business side of health care for a couple of reasons. First, nurses in business can have a big impact on business decisions that will impact patient care. Nurses can help keep the caring possibility alive. Second, we need the nurses who work on the business side of health care to teach and influence nurses who work in patient care. They can help us learn ways to contribute to cost-containment efforts, and help us to realize that, in the end, being fiscally sound is, in itself, a part of caring for our patients and our society.

As our society grapples with bringing health care costs down, there has been great debate about the terms "managed competition" and "managed care." Inglehard (1994) describes managed competition as dividing up physicians and hospitals into competing economic units called "accountable health care partnerships" that would contract with insurance purchasing cooperatives to provide standardized packages of medical benefits at a fixed rate per capita.

Inglehard believes that economic incentives are the principle determinant of how patients, payers, and providers behave when they seek or render medical care. That seems a little callous to me. I do not believe that economics are the only motivator. I have seen all of these groups make exceptions to their sometimes strict policies for the good of individuals. Reinhardt (1994) defines "managed competition" as a highly structured and highly regulated system that forces vertically integrated, income-seeking managed-care systems to compete for patients on the basis of prepared "capitation premiums."

Another term being used is "managed care." Inglehard (1994) defines "managed care" as a system that integrates the financing and delivery of medical care by contracts with selected physicians and hospitals to furnish a comprehensive set of health care services to enrolled members for a preset monthly premium (referred to as "capitation"). Managed care has strong utilization review and quality controls and financial incentives for

A Caring Approach in Nursing Administration

the patient to use only the plan's facilities. Reinhardt (1994) defines managed care as external monitoring of ongoing doctor-patient relationships to make sure that physicians prescribe only "appropriate" interventions. Reinhardt wrote that American proponents of managed competition and managed care believe that, by paying for everything that is beneficial but denying payment for everything else, the nation can avoid setting arbitrary global budgets and will, in the end, devote the "right" percentage of the GNP to health care. Instead, Reinhardt says that the health services industry will continue to grow but the clinical freedom, as older Americans once knew it, will be all but dead.

Managed care is the basic system behind HMOs. There has been great hope and excitement about HMOs in the past decade. Initially, they were thought to have great savings as opposed to fee-for-service medicine. Some people still believe that HMOs are the only way to get a handle on health care costs. But in recent reports, the costs of providing care in HMO hospitals were, in some cases, higher than regular hospitals. Part of the reason for the change is that, in the beginning, the HMOs recruited young, healthy people, thus holding costs down. As their populations have aged, they have had to provide more care to their members. Also, other hospitals have changed their way of doing business. There is less altruism and more attention to the bottom line. They are addressing inefficiency, duplication, excessive overhead, and overcapacity. Yet all the systems we try leave holes in the provision of health care to our citizens. The Select Committee on Aging of the United States House of Representatives said: "When millions are forced to seek charity for whatever health care they need, a nation can feel no pride in having the best care in the world" (p. 99).

Anders (1996) wrote about the advent and progress of HMOs. By the end of the 1980s, there was tremendous frustration throughout our American society about the astronomical increase in the cost of health care.

The most desperate group was employers. History had led employees to expect employers to pay all their health insurance as a part of their salary/benefit package. But health insurance became so expensive that employers had to insist that employees pay part of their health care out of their pocket. It was thought that, if people had to pay for even a little of their health care bills, they would cut down on the use of medical services, thus lowering the costs of health care. That was a very unpopular decision, but all other efforts at cost containment (second surgical opinions and switching as many things as possible to outpatient status) had failed. In the United States, there had been twenty-five years of business frustration with the mounting costs of health care. Insurance had evolved haphazardly with no central control. There was growing confidence in American capitalism and dwindling support of government programs.

Managed care and HMOs amounted to a power grab by employers and insurance companies. While espousing quality care as important, the managed care programs' goals were first and foremost cost-containment measures. The basic strategy of managed care and the ensuing HMOs was that a set amount of money would be collected each year for each enrollee. Then these systems would pay doctors and hospitals a negotiated fee for the service received. If the hospital or HMOs spent less money than the premiums, they could keep the extra money as profit. If, however, they spent more than what they were paid, the HMO would assume the loss. And so, the whole goal of health providers changed from "more treatment resulted in more money," to one where "less service means more money."

One of the first HMOs was Kaiser Permanente, which was started in the 1940s. While it was cost effective, it had a poor reputation from other doctors who considered the HMO doctors as "selling out to big business" and as those who "couldn't make it in private practice."

In the 1970s, President Nixon embraced HMOs and passed a law requiring all businesses with over twenty-five employees to offer an HMO alternative for its employees. By the 1990s, almost every part of American health care had been affected by the influence of HMOs. A new elite rose to power—administrators, statisticians, and doctors who could generate and understand computer-generated data, which allowed them to reduce costs. Practicing physicians were given bonuses if they performed efficiently and reprimanded if they were not efficient.

Another factor of HMOs that has tarnished their reputation is the financial picture of its executives. In large HMO systems, executives are paid over $1 million per year salaries; with other bonuses and stock options adding up to a total yearly income of $15 million. These executives see themselves as typical successful businessmen/women, but when the public learns of such large salaries, they are angry and frustrated. Many of us in the public want health care to be a benevolent system where huge profits should not be given to executives and shareholders.

A Caring Approach in Nursing Administration

Large HMOs have merged and taken over or bought many smaller hospitals. Anders says that some of the huge conglomerates have so much money that they don't know how to spend it all. Traditionally, all the "profit" in not-for-profit systems went back into providing patient care. Over 90 percent of the money that was paid in to the organization went back into patient care. Anders reports that now the for-profit organizations are putting only 68 percent to 78 percent of income back into direct patient care services. The rest of the money is going to executives, administration, and shareholders. For those of us who have worked in patient care for many years, it is devastating to see patient care resources shrink to a level that sometimes feel unsafe while the executives live in luxury.

The executives in the HMOs often embrace "total quality management," which looks at statistics, and expect their organization to run like a factory. HMOs have good records for preventive care. They look at statistics such as the number of children being inoculated, women getting mammograms, and other cancer screening, which are impressive. The problem comes when someone gets sick; the HMOs' executives have no expertise in the treatment of sick people. HMOs try *never* to focus on individual cases gone bad. They are willing to let some problems go by so they can focus on impersonal cost analysis. The executives never get exposed to patients, so the executives' concern is the wallet and the bottom line. Cost cutting affects the entire organization. Of particular concern to us is that direct care providers are cut and cut, leaving many nurses to feel they have no time to be caring.

The moral justification for health care executives is a belief that good health care can be achieved at lower cost. Sometimes the HMOs put so much energy into cost cutting that the mission actually becomes to make as much money as possible. They are happy when doctors order fewer tests, when patients are discharged from hospitals as quickly as possible, and when not every request for specialists is approved. They often do not even give a thought to the effects of such decisions on people needing care. While these cost-minimizing measures may be good for running efficiently, the system is not set up to emphasize quality of care. It is not impossible to be caring in these systems, as I believe every nurse chooses caring with each patient interaction. But with systems that are so bureaucratic, I think nurses will have to have a loud voice to move HMOs toward a caring philosophy.

HMOs are able to cut costs because they are large enough to negoti-ate deep discounts with hospitals, doctors, pharmacies, labs, and x-ray facilities. The HMOs can become so absurd that patients must run all around town trying to use the covered services. I have been admitted to a covered hospital but found that some services (lab, x-rays, anesthesiolo-gists) are not covered. There have been documented cases of people dying while being transported to HMO-covered emergency rooms when they could have been saved if they had gone to the closest ER.

The issue of choice is perhaps the most fundamental problem with HMOs. The patient is given a list of primary-care doctors (sometimes the list is long and sometimes it is very short). Then the patient has to get referrals from their primary-care doctor before going to any specialist. All of the HMO doctors are expected to give as few referrals as possible, and the specialists are instructed to give as little care as possible. These prac-tices produce loss of trust between patients and providers. Patients and families no longer feel certain that their doctor is making an all-out effort to help them. This automatically diminishes the trust between patient and physicians, and sometimes the nurse is left to deal with the distrustful patient. For someone like me who has had the same primary-care physi-cian for many years, changing doctors is very frightening and traumatic. In my case, we have some decision-making power in choosing an HMO, so we chose the HMO that our doctors belong to. The system is not car-ing, but the nurses can remain the caring connection.

HMOs are best at treating routine illnesses where care can be stan-dardized and minimized. The areas of weakness are heart disease, cancer, emergency care, mental health, chronic disease, and the frail elderly (Anders, 1996). The more complex a case gets, the less control the HMOs can exert, and the more pressure is put on the providers of care. It can be very frustrating and difficult for the patients, the nurses, and the physi-cians. Anders found one study where a doctor was hired by HMOs to investigate quality of care in their organizations. The doctor found that primary-care physicians did not recognize crucial symptoms and special-ists were not consulted in time. He concluded that HMOs "simply aren't providing the smart guidance and oversight they espouse" (p. 228).

Teisberg, Porter, and Brown (1994) also wrote about managed care. They say that, during the decade following diagnostic related groupings (DRGs), the average length of stay for hospitalized patients decreased by

A Caring Approach in Nursing Administration

50 percent and the number of patients hospitalized decreased by 20 percent. It certainly does appear that the payers and HMOs are already reforming the health care system. These authors point out that denying claims, which is a highly touted cost-cutting method, doesn't really do anything to bring costs down at all. It just shifts the cost from the insurance company to the doctors, hospitals, and patients.

In years gone by, insurance companies were advocates for patients, but now the insurance companies are adversarial to patients. The compassion of the past has become merely a cost, so the goal of the insurer is to *deny* benefits.

I was recently hospitalized for eight days. I was very sick and it took some time to diagnose and treat me. We had just changed insurance companies, and I was shocked when they denied coverage for the whole hospitalization for "lack of clinical information." That meant that I had to call all my doctors to get information, and I was still bedridden and very sick. After weeks of waiting, the insurance company agreed to pay all but two days of my hospital stay. But it was a terrible frustration and worry at a time when I didn't need to be hassled. I think disallowing the two days was a message—we're in charge, and you better not use any services. Certainly, I did not feel cared for.

In a managed-care situation (my insurance company was an HMO), the patient has no choices. It becomes the responsibility of the employer to consider costs and quality when choosing an insurance company for its employees. Many employers are just looking for the cheapest policy they can find, but as employees begin to complain about their insurance coverage, I think many companies will listen to employees and began to demand quality care instead of just cheap care.

Teisberg, Porter, and Brown say that the cost cutting of HMOs has had some good effects. Health care has been examined and examined, and some of the savings have been very positive. The providers, however, have had to deal with more and more insurance companies systems. There are about 1,500 insurance companies in the country and about 200 companies in any local area. They are, as I have said, not caring in nature. For example, the cost cuttings have not really reduced costs. When insurance companies refuse to pay for services, it just switches the costs to the hospitals who does not get paid, or to the patient, who must pay for the costs. Another fact that is not examined closely is the figures on decreasing health care. The costs have not really gone down, they are just increasing at a rate that is slower than expected. Costs are still going up faster in health care than is the GNP, but the increases are now 6–9 percent instead of the 12–26 percent that we had in the past. The anticipation of reform has already had an impact, but Teisberg, Porter, and Brown believe that we still will need a systematic introduction of clear competitive market incentives that could achieve dramatic results.

It is an important time for nurses and admitting people to be as caring as possible. The first contact for patients is usually with these people. When I was so sick, I found a lady who worked for one of my doctors. She was very caring, and I knew I could call her any time. I also met several nurses who made me feel cared for and cared about.

So, again, we find instances of caring, but not a caring system. It is important for there to be public discussion about changing health care. Teisberg, Porter, and Brown suggest that public policy is needed in order to adequately change the health care system. They believe that some consolidation is good to decrease capacity, but excessive consolidation will risk creating a few very powerful providers who may not feel the need to keep competitive or to continue searching for new treatments and medications.

Patients and families are finally starting to speak out about the failures of HMOs. In our city, people are going to the press about their problems, and they are also starting to sue and receive huge judgments. Employers also are feeling concerned about the lack of service their HMOs are giving, and they can play a major role in improving the health care system. They will demand that low costs are maintained, but they will keep track of how employees feel about their HMOs. Regulators can also do much to hold HMOs to higher standards. For example, in our state a legislative committee was formed to examine and make suggestions about the treatment of intractable pain. I was on the committee, and was surprised and pleased to see three bills pass through the legislative process. One of the bills requires managed-care companies to provide treatment for patients with intractable pain. I belong to a chronic-pain support group, and the new law has allowed two of our members to get treatment by pain specialists.

Anders (1996) also feels that, as HMOs get bigger and more dominant, there may be only a few huge HMOs that will dictate to the whole

A Caring Approach in Nursing Administration

health care system. But, Anders finds an intriguing development in the consolidation of doctors into large groups (sometimes with hospitals). The question is, "Can doctors become effective businessmen who can negotiate contracts directly with hospitals?" Employers may see an opportunity in working directly with providers to cut out the need for the middleman—the HMOs. Employers could cut overhead costs and ensure that a bigger share of the premiums would go back into patient care services. As Anders suggests:

> Eventually the pioneers of the HMO industry may be viewed much like the corporate raiders of the 1980s—intensely provocative change agents who briefly seized control of a big piece of the economy but faded from the scene as society found a more palatable way of carrying out their mission [in health care, that would be caring]. We are only part way through the cycle. At some point, doctors will figure out how to run a cost effective medical system without abandoning compassion . . . And at that point, the swashbuckling middlemen will be left with much less to do. (p. 262)

Let us think for a moment about how the government is involved in this health care debate. Litman (1994) wrote that it is a truism of American political life that government is only permitted to do that which private institutions either cannot or are unwilling to do. He said that the United States is a system of federalism predicated on a representative government. There is an emphasis on minority rights, majority rules, and preservation of individual liberty. We take our freedom very seriously and are suspicious of established authority.

Government's influence in health care is a well-established fact. Historically, the government has accepted responsibility for the health care of veterans, Indians, the armed forces, public health, facility construction, training grants for health care personnel, funding a majority of health care research, and coverage for the old and poor through Medicare and Medicaid. But federal intervention has often been on an ad hoc basis without an overall plan. It seems like the government has been asked to cover the highest users of health care—the old, the poor, and the disabled. Then, when costs rise, they try to cut down on coverage. That is certainly what has happened with Medicare and Medicaid. The hospitals are being reimbursed at a level lower than actual costs for care, and so hospitals "shift" costs to other paying patients. Now, as insurance companies refuse to cover costs not incurred by their patients, the financial picture for hospitals is shaky.

Lee and Benjamin (1994) wrote that government programs already cover more than 40 percent of health care costs and 65 percent of research and development costs. The government spends more and more and yet its reform role remains halting and limited. Litman (1994) points out that government-run health care programs have been in operation for many years in many countries. Government intervention was established under Bismarck in Germany in 1883 and has been adopted in some form in nearly one-half of the world's population, including most of Europe. These authors note that no modern government could disdain responsibility for the health of its people nor would they wish to do so, but Americans are still very wary of a government health system. Litman says that in the United States, incrementalism, rather than fundamental change, has been the hallmark of federal policies. He and many others feel that the only way a health care system can be fundamentally changed in this country is to maintain a tenuous and strained partnership between the government and the voluntary system.

In the 1940s and 1970s, the government tried to initiate government regulation into the health care system. But when Ronald Reagan was elected president, the whole approach changed. Reagan deregulated the health care system and tried to stimulate procompetitive market forces. Reagan's conservative views led him to minimize the effect of government intervention and encourage the free-market order. His ideology appeals to those wanting authority, allegiance, and tradition, with the family (narrowly defined) as central to maintaining the state. He was staunchly opposed to welfare programs. He dismantled some services such as the neighborhood health clinics and public health services. This approach was continued by President Bush, so we had twelve years to let the free-market system straighten out the health care system. Unfortunately, health care costs continued to climb at all-time high rates, and there has been more criticism of the system than ever.

Bush continued the Reagan strategy of privatization, competition, and deregulation laced with concern about the urgency of cost containment. Just weeks before the election in which Clinton defeated Bush, Bush began talking about the crises in health care, but he really had no plan to deal with it. Estes (1994) notes that during the Reagan-Bush years, costs of health care increased threefold from $250 billion to $870 billion.

Clinton put forward a comprehensive government health care package that would provide health care for all Americans. The major components of the Clinton plan included universal access, a comprehensive benefit package, long-term care, prescription coverage, dental coverage, mental health coverage, and preventive care. He believed in managed competition and in forming huge health alliances that would not be allowed to turn people away because of preexisting conditions. There would be a National Health Board to administer the program. There would be an employer mandate (all employers would have to pay for part of the health insurance for its employees), and everyone would have a National Health Security Card so that their benefits could never be taken away.

I believe the Clinton plan was caring in nature. It would have covered everybody and the coverage was comprehensive. However, there was a great deal of dissatisfaction about the Clinton plan from many sources. Strong lobbies from the doctors, hospitals, and, most vehemently, the insurance companies made Clinton's plan an impossible dream.

Since the Republicans came into power in the Congress in 1994, the health care crisis seems to have taken a back seat to debureaucratization of government. Perhaps the lesson to be learned is that no one political group can change health care: it will take a strong consensus among the people before meaningful change will occur.

The good part of the recent past is that there have been many important technological improvements in health care, so more lives can be saved and suffering diminished. The problem is that we can improve technology almost without limit. But technological improvements are responsible in large part for the increase in costs. Nurses know that every new machine or procedure means more nursing time, not less. Thus the industrial model of substituting machines for people just does not work. Health care is a whirling system of change, but no one can, or will, take measures to slow down technology to cut down on costs. In medicine, we find that there is always more that could be done for every patient, and every patient wants every piece of health care they can get. So the costs get higher while care gets more complex (which may not be as helpful as we think!) and frustration on every front grows and grows. Most policy-makers see very little way out without upsetting a lot of people, and those people vote! The feelings of frustration are so severe that the idea that health care can be caring seems ludicrous. Everyone wants the best health care, but at the same time we do not want it to cost so much. Lee, Soffel, and Luft (1994) list the factors increasing costs as: 1. market failure; 2. technology; 3. administrative costs; 4. unnecessary care and defensive medicine; 5. excess capacity (too many hospital beds and doctors); 6. patient complexity; and 7. productivity.

Ginzberg (1994) believes that the first challenge in health care reform is to impress on all the concerned parties that time is running out and that unless a reform effort begins now, the long-term costs will be horrendous. The goal must be to reduce cost and expand access to health care. Inglehard (1994) quoted President Clinton as saying in 1993:

> All our efforts to strengthen the economy will fail—let me say this again, I feel so strongly about it—all our efforts to strengthen the economy will fail unless we also take this year—not next year, not five years from now, but this year—bold steps to reform our health care system.
>
> (p. 335)

Blumenthal (1994) reminds us that cost control and improved access carry political risks. He writes that politicians will have to feel convinced that the voting public, including a large segment of the middle class, is deeply discontented with the system as it is before they will take action to reform it. Blumenthal believes that any change the government may undertake will be incremental, and will build and preserve the components of the employer-based, private insurance industry, the pluralistic delivery system, fee for service, free choice of doctor, and a strong role for state government. With all these constraints, one wonders how there will be any reform at all. One way to reform is to have a government-run system. But most people think there are just too many interest groups to let that happen. The other extreme is to continue the free-market system, which has proven so problematic, and the third option is to have a combined system where people still have choice, but the government may put caps on costs. Some theorists say that we can have one or the other type of these systems, but the combined system will be the most difficult to keep a handle on. By the next generation, we may have learned that a mixed system is bad in every respect except one: it mirrors our ambivalence.

Lundberg (1994) says we should retain the following characteristics of successful health reform: 1. insure universal access to basic care; 2. produce real cost control; 3. stop self-referral to physician-owned facilities; 4. change the tort system of liability; 5. drastically expand managed care and managed competition; 6. insure that all Americans have a primary care physician; 7. retain a private-public mix of payers; 8. establish global budgeting; 9. limit excess capacity and utilization, and establish limits and ceilings for costs; and 10. establish a national health care expenditure board with independent authority to effect such decisions.

As we look at health reform itself, we should remember that Americans are more dissatisfied with their health care than the Canadians or British. One study showed that 91 percent of Americans called for fundamental change in health care (Lee, Soffel, and Luft, 1994). These authors believe that Americans are especially worried about out-of-pocket expenses. The public attributes high costs to unnecessary tests, overpaid doctors, wasteful hospitals, profiteering drug companies, and greedy malpractice lawyers.

One of the complaints of health care analysts has been that part of the reason costs have increased so much is that consumers do not care about the costs because they do not pay for them directly (the insurance companies do). I believe that this is no longer a valid complaint since the deductibles and copayments are so high. Consumers become more and more frightened as they see their own part of health care costs climbing so rapidly. In fact many people *with* health care insurance feel they have none because they can no longer afford going to the doctor because their own part of the costs is too high. Still, many politicians feel there is no need for fundamental change in health care. Politicians will have to feel convinced that the voting public is deeply discontented before they will act. Clearly President Clinton believed this issue had reached "critical mass" and he committed to major change. The 1994 Congress, however, had a Republican majority, and since their election, I have not heard a word about government changes in health care. I think that health reform will happen and that it will be a mixed system. One of my colleagues suggests that even if the government does nothing, the institutions are already reforming the system in their rush to be ready for reform. My hope for reform is that we obtain universal access and maintain low enough out-of-pocket costs so that people feel free to get health care. There are many other components that should be addressed, but these two have the greatest impact on the system being caring. I hope that nurses can have impact on the final package, and I hope they continue to impose caring values. As we have learned from previous chapters, it will take strong, open leadership to get us to the place where costs are controlled and caring is the norm.

So, how are nurses fairing in this health care debate? Harrington et al. (1994) believe that nurses could indeed be a big part of a more cost-efficient health care system. Nurses have proven their worth in many areas. For example, certified registered nurse anesthetists are the sole providers for obstetrical care in 85 percent of rural hospitals, and provide 65 percent of all anesthesia. These authors believe that nurses could provide as much as 50 percent to 90 percent of ambulatory care needs. They believe that laws should be changed to allow nurses hospital privileges, and that the base rates for services should be based on the services rather on who provides them (historically, nurses got less money than physicians when they performed the same treatments). Recently, in several states, registered nurses have been given prescriptive authority that will enhance their practice. They will no longer have to rely on physicians to approve all drugs they use. These developments are encouraging for nurses who want to try independent nurse roles.

Aiken (1994) believes that nursing is among the important factors that explain variation in death rates between hospitals. She feels that most nurses would say: "I love my work; I hate my job." This, I believe, is a reflection of how important it is for nurses to believe they have the resources to do a good job. Aiken reports that the high turnover in hospital nursing has to do with the decrease in the number of nurses available for direct patient care. In addition, many hospitals have decreased their support services, making more work for nurses to cover. Aiken reports that nurses perceive that staffing levels are dangerously inadequate and that levels of dissatisfaction are high. I personally believe that nurses can be pushed for more productivity (more, sicker patients to care for) to a certain point. At that point, the nurse loses heart and may become angry and bitter. Their work will suffer because they can no longer care. Organizational constraints have pushed him/her away from being able to care, and patient care and organizational harmony are compromised.

Watson (1990) wrote that, if our aim for caring in nursing is higher than achieving machinelike knowledge, it is not enough to be technically correct. Human care, writes Watson, needs to be explicitly incorporated into nursing's meta-paradigm, and our aim should be to express and to reflect life and life forces. To do so we will need nursing leaders who understand caring and its central role in helping patients achieve improvement of their health.

MacPherson (1989) wrote that many nurses are simply leaving their profession or choosing to become nurse entrepreneurs as a means of escaping the alienating conditions within the hospital. If we are to keep good nurses in hospitals, strategies for making caring possible in a corporate world must be developed rapidly by nurses and other health care workers. I believe that we should encourage nurse entrepreneurs, because they will expand what we now see as the health care system, but we must not let hospitals become the place where nurses least want to work.

Fagin (1994) writes that nurses have stopped the nurse-doctor game where the nurse always has to act subservient to the doctor. Many doctors are puzzled and confused and feel betrayed and angry. New models of nursing are being implemented to utilize nurses better and increase their satisfaction. Fagin believes that the knowledge of physicians and nurses give them a lot to share. She says that the extent to which physicians are able to move to a broader, more-shared perspective of nursing, the more they will directly contribute to the satisfaction of nurses, patients, and doctors.

Davis (1988) wrote about the need for nursing to have strong values in relation to health policy. Such values include: 1. belief in the individual's right to health care; 2. belief in humanistic health care; 3. belief in the provision of health care by the best-qualified practitioner; and 4. a strong advocacy role for patients. With a united value system, nursing can be more effective in presenting its positions to, and gaining the support of, the public.

My concern about nursing in regard to health care reform is that we will do too little to impact the changes in the system. We are in a much better position to make our concerns heard in the political arena than ever before because of the increase in nursing organizations. Recently, the first lady, Hillary Clinton, spoke to a group of nurses, emphasizing the potential nurses have in health care now and in the future. It is my fear, however, that all the diverse nursing groups will not pool their influence to make the biggest difference possible.

I believe that the government people trying to devise a new health care system are open to the influence of nursing if we will just raise our voices to be heard. I think it is important that our issues surrounding the health reform debate must be patient-related. So many of the interest groups trying to influence reform are doing so from the standpoint of what they can get for themselves, not what is best for patients. I see potential for collaboration about patient care between physicians and nurses, and think we should pursue alliances based on patient care issues. Nurses as a group with interests of their own can have impact, but so can nurses individually. I have started a writing campaign of my own, and I have received replies from all of our state's senators and representatives. They do not all agree with my position, but they are listening to their constituents very closely on this issue. If all 3 million nurses wrote letters, think of the impact we could have. Perhaps the direction of health care reform will be settled by the time this book is published, and I can only hope that we nurses feel we have had a part in its creation.

Stimpson (1992) wrote about the role of nurse policy analysts. She believes that nurses who pursue the study of health policy should be viewed as subspecialists in nursing just as nurse administrators or clinical nurse specialists are. She wrote that nurses are particularly qualified to assume the role of analyst because of their analytic and communication skills and their health expertise. So far, there are a handful of nurse policy analysts, and we need to have more people in active political roles. The role of the nurse policy analyst is to focus on health care as it occurs both within and out of traditional care-providing institutions. A major function is to provide information to decision makers through the policy analysis process. The nurse analyst must utilize analytical skills to identify related factors and forecast future outcomes. There are many particular roles for this nurse from everything to being a "staffer" in Washington to being in an elected or appointed government position. While having nurse policy analysts is exciting, each nurse is responsible for keeping up to date on health care issues. Nurses know very personally what the health care system puts people through. As we reform the system, nurses must play a visible part.

In nursing, we hear some familiar, similar terms: managed care, case management, and others. This is all very confusing to many nurses who have viewed themselves and doctors as managing patient care for many years. It seems like the history of this movement began about fifteen years ago, when costs were going so high so quickly. Our first response was to

A Caring Approach in Nursing Administration

hire discharge planners who would facilitate getting patients out of the hospital as quickly as possible. There was also a strong component to this role that tried to make sure patients received appropriate care at home. Costs continued to rise, so we hired utilization reviewers. Their job was much more restricted to finding ways to cut costs. Physicians were outraged to have nurses and doctors in an office telling them what they should do with their patients. Then the insurance companies decided that hospital personnel could not be trusted to keep costs down, so the insurance utilization reviewers were born. Many nurses have carved out new jobs in the managed-care arena, and I applaud their efforts. Nurses have been very effective case managers in the past, and they fall easily into the new case management roles in hospitals, free-standing health care facilities, and third-party payer systems.

Now the terms "managed care" or "case management" are being thrown around as new nursing models of care within hospital settings. Even within nursing, however, the terms are rarely defined or implemented in the same way. Some hospitals claim great success with such programs, and others fail miserably. In some nursing models, case managers are hired as a new job classification, and they have the authority to tell the staff nurse what to do. In other models, staff nurses are becoming the case managers.

This is all very frustrating to me. I believe that having four or five levels basically doing the same job is ridiculous. If there is a problem with the real case managers (doctors and nurses), then teach them to do things differently—don't hire five levels of bureaucracy to confuse the patient care process and increase administrative costs! In the United States, the administration costs in health care are 25 percent as compared to Canada's 2.5 percent.

This is a classic example of outside pressure causing expenditures on defensive mechanisms, not on correcting the basic problem. As we learned in organizational theory, organizations initially put all their resources into producing their product. As the organization or industry ages, there are more and more pressures from outside. The response is to hire people to defend the organization or industry. In health care's case, we have seriously jeopardized our product by paying more attention to management issues than to issues of our product—patient care. There may be many opportunities for nurses providing primary care to case manage and perhaps some areas are so complicated that they need specific case managers (which used to be the job of clinical nurse practitioners). I just cannot stop thinking about my Magnet Hospital experience where we put all the resources at the bedside and taught the nurses what they needed to know to do their jobs right.

Himali (1995) wrote in *The American Nurse* about managed care. She points out that the original theory of managed care was a good one: patients receive care through a single "seamless" system as they move from wellness to sickness and back to wellness again. In the early days of managed care, the emphasis was on an efficiently run system that stressed continuity of care, a full range of services, prevention, and early intervention. Now, however, for many nurses, managed care has become synonymous with cost-containment efforts that are driving RN layoffs. Himali quotes Anna Gilmore as saying:

> The problem lies not in managed care, but rather in how providers choose to spend the money that managed care plans pay them. In many instances, we see hospitals putting money into capital, new equipment, and increasing the salaries of their chief executive officers, rather than putting it into where it really should be put—and where they are being paid to put it—and that's into providing good quality care to patients while they're in hospitals.
>
> (p. 1)

Managed care has become a quick fix for many hospitals that have financial problems. But Himali suggests that, at some point in managed care, hospitals will be forced to compete not only on the basis of price but on quality as well.

Reinhardt (1994) believes that managed competition and managed care are the last hurrah of the free market. He wrote:

> It is my thesis. . . . Americans most likely will learn that a managed care managed competition approach will do so many wondrous things, but it will not be able to stop the medical arms race that characterizes the American health care system. Sooner or later the U.S. health system will therefore envelope the competing medico-fishbowls by a global national budget imposed from the top. Thus it is my bet that, around the year 2005, the health systems of Canada and Europe, too, will be a combination of budgets and statistical

A Caring Approach in Nursing Administration

medico-fishbowls and that there will be a brisk commerce of ideas among health-services researchers and health care managers across the globe on how best to construct these medico-fishbowls, how best to behold them, and how best to direct the busy medico-fish within them toward desirable ends.

(p. 277)

Vladek (1994) wrote that managed care is supposed to be the grand design for the complete reorganization of the American health care system, but that in fact it is an untested theory about reducing costs. Proponents of managed competition oppose price setting, which, in effect, allows the system to continue to grow unfettered. They support managed care because they do not believe its cost-containment mechanisms will really work, and they are afraid other mechanisms would. It does, however, seem to ignore the central issue that American citizens who get sick cannot get health care because they have no health insurance. Vladek calls that a disgrace! Friedman (1994) agrees, saying that a democracy that thinks of itself as the moral hope of the world cannot justify our grave inequities in health care, which in most countries is considered an essential human right.

This has been a long, twisting chapter to answer the question, "Is the health care system caring?" But a closer look shows that it is not a simple question at all. In all the world, there is not a health care system as complicated as ours, and we are doing our analysis at a confusing time in history.

I guess the best way I can answer the question is to speak of my own experiences as a health care recipient. I have had a severe medical problem for sixteen years, and I have lived the changes in the system. I would have to agree with the nurses that most of the care provided by nurses is caring. I would also say, however, that how caring is delivered depends on the nurse and the hospital. In one hospital, I was checked once postoperatively, and I never saw another nurse until I called for help getting to the bathroom. I was about two hours postoperative, so the nurse did help me get to the bathroom without losing my intravenous setup. However, as soon as I was in the bathroom, she left without saying a word, and never came back to help me get back to the bed. This was in a hospital where I know staffing levels are bad. The nurses I saw showed no enthusiasm for their work. They seemed to be in a state where caring had been lost. In another hospital, I was several hours postop, and my pain level was intolerable. The nurses in this hospital had better staffing levels, and they treated me caringly. However, they were not willing to try anything else or to call the doctor for pain relief until the doctor's order for a pill once every four hours was past. The nurses seemed to have little sense of themselves as decision makers or patient advocates. In the third hospital, the nurses were very caring, and when my pain got out of control, they used other methods of treating the pain and took the initiative to get more medicine ordered. These nurses seemed sure of themselves and spent their time in the patients' rooms. One night, I had no visitors, so my nurse asked someone else to watch her other patients for fifteen minutes and "came to visit me." Recently I was hospitalized again, and I was disappointed with my nursing care, nurse aides did most of my care, and they were just doing tasks. When I saw nurses, they were caring, but they were obviously very busy. Barter, McLaughlin, and Thomas (1997) did a study that found that registered nurses were dissatisfied with the unlicensed assistants who could not perform delegated tasks, had difficulty communicating patient information, and could not provide more time for RNs to do professional nursing activities.

I know that these are four simple instances of patient contact with nurses, but I have learned a lot about health care from being on the patients' side. Patients can tell when the stress is so high that the nurse really does not have time for you, and they appreciate every minute of contact they have with their nurse. The nurse is the key to their whole hospital (or clinic or some other setting) experience. The doctors are very important, too, and I have had mostly very caring physicians, but they are only there for a few minutes a day. It is the nurse who makes the patient feel really cared for or not.

As for the health care system, I have very little good to say. The good changes that have occurred include prettier rooms, slightly better food, home care, and some sense that you, the patient, are important. In that respect, the system feels more caring. The switch to outpatient treatment has its good and bad parts. It is nice to go home soon, but I will never forget one day when I was sent home in what I thought was too fast a time frame. The biggest problem was that I could hardly make it to the bathroom by myself, and I was left alone all day. With quick discharge, it is important to prepare the patient so he/she can arrange to have help. That is not always easy, since families can rarely take time off to care for you. Coming home prematurely does not feel caring.

The biggest problem area for the patient is in dealing with "the system" when you don't even know who or what that is. My last outpatient testing experience was not a good one. I was told to came to the hospital at 11:30 a.m. for a test that would take a few hours. I was told that I could not drive myself home, so I arranged to have someone pick me up at 3:30, thinking that was plenty of time. Imagine my chagrin when 2 p.m. came along and I had not even been taken down for my test. I knew I had to have a blood test and an IV started, but that certainly did not take three hours. In this situation, it was clearly the convenience of the hospital that took precedence over the convenience of the patient. At another hospital where I had outpatient surgery, I went in a day early and had all my tests done in an efficient manner, and it made me feel that my time was important to them as well as me.

The worst thing of all is the paperwork. At each hospital, I was asked the same questions over and over. After awhile, my husband remarked, "Don't they ever talk to each other? They have it all written down three times." But the whole hospital experience cannot begin to compare with the insurance system. They have *definitely* become less caring. The precertification process can take weeks, and once again they seem to ask the same questions over and over. First, you call them; then they call your doctor; then they may or may not call you back. Usually I have to call them several times to find out what is going on. They drill me about all my medical history, and you feel like it is a test you have to take. If you make it through that procedure, and you get your treatment, you think all is well. Guess again! The worst part is about to hit—getting the bills paid. It seems that no bill gets paid the first time, and usually the hospital or doctor is hassling you for the money because the insurance company is so slow. Then you find out just how big those deductibles and copayments really are. In addition, the insurance company has probably negotiated a discounted fee, and then the provider tries to collect the balance from you. Does this sound caring? It sure does not feel that way. In the good old days of Blue Cross paying all your bills, you at least could recover from whatever ailed you. Now I have to worry about what doctor I can go to and whether it is worth the hassle to have a mammogram. I feel that, since I need medical services, I am the enemy! It feels like the insurance company does everything in its power to keep you from using the benefits you need and deserve. Pretty soon, if you need ongoing care, you begin to wonder if your life is really worth it since the insurance company does not seem to think so.

So, how can we make the system more caring in a time when more and more regulation is on the way? I think it is important to buffer the patient from the hassles as much as possible. I am very much in favor of having a few big insurance companies who will hopefully figure out more simple systems for the patients. I appreciate all the aesthetic improvements in the facilities, but I would tell you to take it all down if it means that my nurses will be too hassled to care for me. Listen to my perspective and create systems that minimize redundancy and wasted time. And once—just once—I wish that someone would recognize what all the health care means to me. Recognize that my illness imposed itself on me, and do not show me blame. Speak to me about what my illness means to my life, and give me all the gentleness and warm smiles you can muster— from the hospital, the nurses and doctors, and, yes, even the dreaded insurance company. Find your own way of influencing health care in a way that keeps the caring alive, for your own sake and for your patients'.

References

Aiken, L. H. (1994). Charting the future of hospital nursing. In Lee and Estes, eds., *The Nation's Health*. Boston: Jones, Barlett Publishers, pp. 177–187.

Anders, G. (1996). *Health Against Wealth: HMOs and the Breakdown of Medical Trust*. Boston, New York: Houghton Mifflin.

Barter, M., F. E. McLaughlin, and S. A. Thomas (1997). Registered nurse role changes and satisfaction with unlicensed assistive personnel. *Journal of Nursing Administration* 27 (1): 29–38.

Blumenthal, D. (1994). The timing and course of health reform. In Lee and Estes, eds., *The Nation's Health*. Boston: Jones, Barlett Publishers, pp. 219–223.

Davis, G. (1988). Nursing values and health care policy. *Nursing Outlook* 36 (6): 289–292.

Eddy, D. (1994). Clinical decision making: From theory to practice. In Lee and Estes, eds., *The Nation's Health*. Boston: Jones, Barlett Publisher, pp. 315–321.

Estes, C. (1994). Privatization, the welfare state, and aging: The Reagan-Bush legacy. In Lee and Estes, eds., *The Nation's Health*. Boston: Jones, Barlett Publishers.

Fagin C. M. (1994). Collaboration between nurses and physicians: No longer a choice. In Lee and Estes, eds., *The Nation's Health*. Boston: Jones, Barlett Publishers, pp. 315–321.

Feeney, A. (1994). Health inequalities and social class. In Lee and Estes, eds., *The Nation's Health*. Boston: Jones, Barlett Publishers.

Friedman, E. (1994). The uninsured: From dilemma to crisis. In Lee and Estes, eds., *The Nation's Health*. Boston: Jones, Barlett Publishers, pp. 302–309.

Fuchs V. C. (1988). The "competition revolution" in healthcare. *Health Affairs* (Summer): 5–25.

Ginzberg, E. (1994). Health care reform: Where are we and where should we be going? In Lee and Estes, eds., *The Nation's Health*. Boston: Jones, Barlett Publishers, pp. 314-318.

Harrington, C., S. L. Feetham, P. A. Moccia, and G. R. Smith (1994). Health care access: Problems and policy recommendations. In Lee and Estes, eds., *The Nation's Health*. Boston: Jones, Barlett Publishers.

Himali, U. (1995). Managed care: Does the promise meet the potential? *The American Nurse* (June): 1, 12, 14, 16.

Inglehard, J. K. (1994). Managed competition. In Lee and Estes, eds., *The Nation's Health*. Boston: Jones, Barlett Publishers, pp. 231–237.

Lee P. L. and A. E. Benjamin (1994). Health policy and politics of health care. In Lee and Estes, eds., *The Nation's Health*. Boston: Jones, Barlett Publishers, pp. 121–137.

Lee, P. R. and C. Estes, eds., (1994). *The Nation's Health*. Boston: Jones, Bartlett, Publishers.

Lee, P. R., D. Soffel, and H. S. Luft (1994). Costs and coverage: Pressures toward health care reform. In Lee and Estes, eds., *The Nation's Health*. Boston: Jones, Barlett Publishers.

Litman, T. J. (1994). Government and health: the political aspects of health care: a sociopolitical overview. In Lee and Estes, eds., *The Nation's Health*. Jones, Bartlett Publishers.

Lundberg, G. D. (1994). National health care reform: The aura of inevitability intensifies. In Lee and Estes, eds., *The Nation's Health*. Boston: Jones, Bartlett Publishers, pp. 238–241.

MacPherson, K. I. (1989). A new perspective on nursing and caring in a corporate context. *Advances in Nursing Science* 11 (4): 32–39.

McKeown, T. (1994). Determinants of health. In Lee and Estes, eds., *The Nation's Health*. Boston: Jones, Barlett Publisher, pp. 6–13.

Ray, M. A. (1989). The theory of bureaucratic caring for nursing practice in the organizational culture. *Nursing Administration Quarterly* 13 (2): 31–42.

Reinhardt, U. (1994) Providing access to health and controlling costs: The universal dilemma. In Lee and Estes, eds., *The Nation's Health*. Boston: Jones, Barlett Publishers, pp. 238–241.

———. (1986). Rationing the healthcare surplus: An American tragedy. *Nursing Economics* 4 (3): 101–108.

Relman, A. S. (1994). The health care industry: Where is it taking us? In Lee and Estes, eds., *The Nation's Health*. Boston: Jones, Bartlett Publisher, pp. 263–278.

Rice, D. P. (1994). Health status and national health priorities. In Lee and Estes, eds., *The Nation's Health*. Boston: Jones, Barlett Publishers, pp. 45–58.

Select Committee on Aging, U.S. House. (1994). Medicare and Medicaid's 25th anniversary—much promised, accomplished, and left unfinished. In Lee and Estes, eds., *The Nation's Health*. Boston: Jones, Barlett Publisher, pp. 94–99.

Shore, M. F. and H. Levinson (1986). Sounding board on business and medicine. *The New England Journal of Medicine* 313 (5): 319–321.

Stimpson, M. (1992). Nurse policy analyst. *Nursing and Health Care* 12 (1): 10–15.

Teisberg, E. O., M. E. Porter, and G. B. Brown (1994). Making competition in health care work. *Harvard Business Review* 17 (4): 131–141.

Torrens, P. R. and J. Williams (1994). Understanding the present, planning for the future. In Lee and Estes, eds., *The Nation's Health*. Boston: Jones, Barlett Publisher, pp. 59–66.

Vladeck, B. C. (1994). Old snake oil in new bottles. In Lee and Estes, eds., *The Nation's Health*. Boston: Jones, Bartlett Publishers, pp. 279–284.

Watson, J, (1990). Caring knowledge and informed moral passion. *Advances in Nursing Science* 13 (1): 15–24.

CHAPTER SEVEN

Caring and Nursing Economics

After a chapter that focuses on the health care system and current fiscal concerns, it is important for us to follow up with a chapter on economics so that we can understand more completely what is happening in our cost-conscious industry.

My own background in economics includes business courses and reading business literature and the minimal material focusing on economics in nursing. Although I have become right-brained in relation to my caring ideals, I also have an active left-brained appreciation for the numbers, logic, and finite concepts of economics. I learned budgeting as most nurse administrators do: by going through the process. But I learned about the values and procedures of economic control from texts and teachers.

Actually, after my first experience with the budget process, I was hooked. I enjoyed tallying the numbers and determining what they meant. It was clear to me that nursing's power within the organization was directly related to performance in the budgeting process.

In my years as a consultant, I have included budget analysis in almost all my projects. I think the economics of nursing have a lot to do with opportunities for change and creativity. I find many nurse executives to be weak in finances. I remember how dumb I felt at the start of my administration. I studied hard, though, and before long, I could understand the financial officer's lingo. Soon, I had questions he had trouble answering. I found I needed to pull back a bit because of the political ramifications, but I had learned a very important lesson: never let anyone outside of nursing know more about your finances than you do. Knowledge is power, and in today's cost-conscious world, I believe nursing needs to clearly understand its economics.

This chapter is, without a doubt, the most difficult to write. There are so many details about budgeting and economics that it could go on and on. But I want to focus on economic values because that is where caring is considered. For the past eight years, I have been studying economics and wrestling with the terrible dilemma of how to address the issue of economics within a caring framework. I must confess at the outset that I have not come up with any great revelations about it. But I have some ideas about how economics and caring can coexist. It is too important to ignore, anyway, so we will try to come up with some picture of today's economic issues and how they may affect caring.

Economics can be defined in a variety of ways. Cleland (1990) defined economics as a science of choices from scarce or limited resources. Hailstones (1984) defined economics as thriftiness or implementing a budget, as in a household. Thaker (1983) defined "economics as the social science that studies human behavior in response to the necessity of allocating scarce resources among alternative possible uses." However it is defined, the word economics brings thoughts of money and prices.

It is interesting to me that economists define themselves as human scientists. I usually think of them as number-crunchers stuck in an office somewhere just waiting to come after me with a stick because I went "over budget." I saw nothing human about it! But when it comes right down to it, someone has to make up the budget, and it really is not so scientific at all. This view of economics is called "normative economics." Foster (1987) described normative economics as welfare economics that attempts to say what should be rather than what is. It must ultimately rest on some value system. It cannot be entirely "scientific" in the sense of being based entirely on facts that have been verified by careful observation. Foster says that there is a broad consensus about the value system among economists, and it is based on the principle of consumer sovereignty. In that value system, the customer is always right. This is difficult in health care when

A Caring Approach in Nursing Administration

patients sometimes lack the knowledge or capacity to made decisions about their health care. That is why, in health care, it is imperative that the physicians and nurses work closely with the patient or family to make proper choices for the patient. So, on an individual level, consumer sovereignty means making the right decision, medically and financially. There is, however, another level of consumer sovereignty—that of consumers as a whole. The health care system must consider what is best for consumers as a whole. The problem is that "health care" is an indefinable entity, and there is no mechanism to make such decisions. Thus, consumer sovereignty can create conflict between what is best for each patient and what is best for patients as a whole. Economists in health care organizations generally think it is good for all patients to keep the organization alive and fiscally sound. So, when budget time comes around, the financiers will see the good of the organization as supreme. There is little understanding that, if you don't have staff to deliver good care, the health of the organization may be harmful to the health care system as a whole. A few years ago, it was assumed that many hospitals would go broke because of the DRG system. In reality, few hospitals have closed, but many are on the verge of closing or merging with stronger institutions. In fact, it may be economically and qualitatively best for the general population to have some organizations close. The nurses' position economically should be one of austerity without losing the caring element. Nurse executives must find the fine line of what can be cut from the budget without cutting caring. It can be seen as an impossible job, or as an important opportunity. Russell (1986) identified the fundamental dilemma of balancing cost and quality in health care. "Cost containment means giving up at least a little quality. Resources now lag noticeably behind opportunities to use them. Each opportunity must be judged more carefully. The balancing of cost and quality is the balancing of cost against health outcomes" (p. 55).

Schroeder (1993) refers to past economics in health care as "cost unconscious." Neither providers or consumers had incentives to curb costs. Nurses have been buried in the institution's costs with no one really knowing or being responsible for managing nursing resources. Most nurses have recognized they can no longer practice in a traditional cost-unconscious manner and remain members of a viable profession. There are some sites where nursing has been successful financially. Schroeder mentions a nurse-managed clinic for HIV patients that saved about

$1.7 million in two years by keeping patients out of hospitals and providing outpatient treatment. Schroeder says that we need legislative, financial, and professional reforms to use advanced nurse practitioners better.

I agree with Schoeder that we need to continue to press for reforms, but I think nurses have been very involved in finances at the administrative level for the last decade. I agree that nursing should be separated from the room rate, but I do not think nurse administrators have been "cost unconscious." Actually, I think nurses have done a better job of controlling costs than most hospital departments. What amazes me is that the health care administrative costs have been allowed to escalate 300 percent faster than direct care costs.

When the budgets are made up, someone is imposing their view of what should be. For example, the budgets in most hospitals today are made up by the top-level managers, and that usually includes the nurse executive. The primary goal of the nurse administrator is to protect the resources needed for delivery of caring nursing. He/she is not the only one with an economic agenda. I found it particularly difficult when nursing costs were cut to buy a new x-ray machine, and that seemed to happen every year. The budget participants sit down with all the financial data from the year before, the goals of the next year, and about a million requests from managers for more money for programs or equipment. Who gets what approved depends, to some extent, on the values of the administrators making the budget. This is why it is so important to have knowledgeable nurse executives who are strong and willing to assert caring values.

The components of the budget are: 1. volume and revenue projections; 2. the capital budget; 3. the manpower budget; 4. the supply and expense budget; and 5. net revenue expectation. Each piece must be carefully analyzed so that all the pieces come together at the end.

The volume and revenue projections are calculated first. Basically, it involves determining how many patients (outpatient and/or inpatient) you had last year and making predictions about whether they will go up or down. All sources of revenue are then projected. For the only way to know how much you can spend is to know how much money will be coming into the organization. Often, the next step is for the board of directors to make a decision on how much net revenue or profit is expected. In nonprofit organizations, profit is called "reserves" which is the amount of money available for unexpected financial needs. The difference in for-profit and not-for-profit status is that, in not-for-profit organizations, all of the money earned goes back into the organization. In for-profit organizations, profit is taken for shareholders and there is then less money that goes back into the organization. Now we know how much money we expect and how much of a profit is to be made, so the rest of the income can be divided up for the rest of the budget.

The next thing to throw a monkey wrench into the process is the capital budget. With so much new technology coming out every year and every doctor wanting his own specialist's equipment, the requests for capital dollars are usually huge. Sometimes the whole revenue picture can change and profit expectations be lowered to accommodate the capital budget.

We have not yet started on the bread and butter of the budget yet: that is, "How much money do we have to spend on the actual running of the institution?" Usually there is a great deal of pressure to keep the *operating budget* low in order to maximize the money for capital and profit levels. The operating budget is made up of manpower and supply and expense budgets. Some organizations just look at the last year's expenses and project them forward, but that is very dangerous. For one thing, it rewards bad fiscal managers by continuing to give them whatever they used before. For another thing, the next year may be very different than the last. It is best to have the managers make a careful assessment of what business changes they expect and then channel money to where the biggest increases in expenses will be.

The really tough part of the budgeting process for nursing is the manpower budget. Most of the costs of nursing are labor costs, and the units of measure are hours or nursing costs per patient-day. Again, different hospitals use different methods of determining manpower budgets. Some just project from last year's costs and assume that the next year will be the same. Some use a set patient-nurse ratio, and the more sophisticated organizations include the factor of acuity when projecting manpower dollars. In years past, nursing had little leverage to get needed increases in their manpower budgets. Now, patient classification systems can document where patients' needs have increased, and more manpower dollars can be allocated to units documenting changing patient needs.

Patient classification systems have come and gone in some hospitals. I developed one in 1979 that was used for about ten years (I do not know what has been used since). I know the criticisms of patient classification systems, including the complaint that they take into account only nursing tasks. But ours included a place to indicate teaching and counseling needs. Now I would add a place to check off caring treatments. It is important that one not allow some management engineer to talk you into classifying the tasks in order of who can do them. Unless you want all aids doing all baths, etc., your staffing matrix must determine who can do what, not your patient classification system. The system can be configured in many ways, and it should be revised every year or two. I know they are not perfect, but they are a quantitative tool that administrators can understand. We used ours to help us decide which units needed more nursing-care hours based on the patients' needs, not just a head count. It was very helpful.

After you have adjusted for acuity, the nurse administrator must consider not just how much it *has* cost, but also how much it *will* cost in the future. What factors will change in the next year that will increase or decrease nursing costs? For example, implementation of some of the caring modalities may cost more money for the nursing manpower budget, even though the modalities may have an overall savings to the hospital or clinic as patients feel better and need less-expensive technical therapies.

The priorities for budget allocation may include:

1. Maintenance of program activities.

2. Improved productivity or efficiency.

3. Employee compensation.

4. New services.

5. Enhanced technologies.

6. Plant maintenance.

7. Aesthetic upgrades.

8. Increased profit.

There are usually many opinions about which of these priorities are most important. Sometimes compromise will be needed where, for example, one of two new services will be funded to allow for increased employee compensation. It takes an open, flexible management team to come away from the budget process intact.

Once the budget is hammered out (no small feat), all the hospital departments are given their budgets and the budget variance reporting begins. That means that every month the budget comes out, and if one manager is over budget, a justification must be made for any overage, and administration decides if further action is needed.

That is the process behind the budget, but what are the values that determine the budget, and where do they come from? The most basic economic values come from our understanding of economic systems.

The basic understanding of economics is based on the concept of scarcity. This assumes that there is an unlimited desire for goods or services, and that some system has to be in place to decide who gets how much of what. The two systems that dominate economics around the world are capitalism and socialism. While we cannot do an in-depth analysis of the two, a general description can help us understand health care economics.

When we think of capitalism, we immediately think of the United States. Our country was based on the values of individual freedom, and that fits well with capitalism. In a capitalistic society, we usually think of ownership and self-interest, for the basis of capitalism is individual accumulation of wealth. Businesses have the freedom to carry on business however they want. There is limited governmental control, and market competition, with its pricing and selling systems, dominates.

Socialism, however, has a much less positive image to Americans. This system also relies on the concept of scarcity where there are unlimited desires for goods but limited amounts of goods and services. The difference is that in a socialistic system, there is strong central control and ownership. The goal for socialistic systems is equal distribution of goods and services to everyone. Neither system is either all good or all bad, and most systems usually contain elements of both. Now that the Soviet Union has collapsed, there is a clamor around the world for all nations to have a capitalistic economic system. To me, this is very strange, because in our own country we have a mixture of socialism and capitalism. To me, the thing we should be most interested in, when it comes to other countries, is the freedom of their people. I think that freedom is an example of a caring concept in economics. I am more interested in the people and their choices than what system of economics they chose to use. Some people feel that you cannot have freedom with socialism, but the Soviet Union was not the only socialist country in the world. One country that has many socialistic programs is Sweden, where the standard of living and the freedom of its people is strong.

The question we must ask in this book is, "Is health care capitalistic or socialistic, and is that the way we want it to be?" The answer to the question is that health care in this country is a mixture of the two. Remember that the goal in a socialistic system is equal distribution of goods to everyone. Does everyone in our country have equal access to health care? Of course not, but there is a huge debate going on in Congress about whether we should have health care for all Americans. Even in our capitalistic society, we hold fast to the rights of equality for our people. We do not want our people to starve, so we have welfare. And most people believe that everyone should have access to health care. The question is, how do we do that?

In the 1980s and 1990s we tried to run our health care system more capitalistically, and the results were very disheartening to many. It was thought that the costs of health care would come down if we put some price incentives in place. One problem with that was that we already had the socialistic system of Medicare and Medicaid in place. Prices were put on patient care under the diagnostic related groupings (DRG) system. The prices soon were inadequate for the standard of care Americans expect, however, and so the singular action of trying to make health care more capitalistic was a dismal failure. Maybe it would have worked if the prices were higher, but the whole idea was that a capitalistic system would lower costs. The other way it might have worked is if we could have drastically cut health care costs. But no one had the authority to cut costs of utilities or supplies or new technology. So costs continued to go up, and the government did not raise the prices to cover the costs, putting many health care systems in trouble. Patient care was placed in jeopardy, and thus the ideal of caring was in danger of being cut right out of the very difficult budgets.

Within the capitalist system there are different market models. The most pure are the monopoly and the free-market competition systems. In pure competition, there are a large number of producers selling goods and services to knowledgeable consumers who make choices based on the quality, product variation, and price. An example of such a system would be the automobile industry. The other extreme is the monopoly, where there is only one seller of the good or service. An example of this system would be public utilities (although even this industry is now subject to some competition).

In hospitals we have some monopolies and some competition. For example, I read recently that one company is now making 95 percent of all hospital beds. That would allow that company to pretty much charge what they want in a monopolistic fashion. The capitalistic example might be the drug companies that have thousands of drugs, some of which do the very same thing. You can see that in the capitalistic system money must be spent on salesmen and advertising to get doctors to prescribe a particular company's drugs. There is price competition, which tends to drive prices down to get people to buy their goods.

There are also some market models that combine competition and monopoly. One is the monopolistic competition, where many producers sell a somewhat differentiated product in a competitive manner. The other is the oligopoly, where there are a few producers, each one dependent to some extent on the actions and reactions of the others.

In the past, hospitals were thought of as oligopolies because, in any geographic region, there are a limited number of hospitals who can cooperate to keep price competition to a minimum. In small towns, the hospital usually is a monopoly. In cities, there is more competition, but through associations and informal channels, hospitals used to keep prices from fluctuating too much.

The oligopolistic health care system was a comfortable one for health care providers, who were essentially in strong control of their industry. Traditional health care payment systems had responded to the noncompetitive environment by passively reimbursing health care providers whatever it cost to provide care deemed appropriate by physicians. The incentive for health care providers was to provide as much service as possible, since more service automatically meant more revenue.

The economics of health care have changed rapidly the past fifteen years from an oligopoly to a more free-market approach. This has occurred in both the government and private sectors. In the 1970s, the government leaned toward heavily regulating health care by initiating comprehensive planning boards. Costs continued to climb. In the 1980s, attitudes about health care costs took a new twist. Rather than regulating costs, the government tried to do the opposite by introducing a free-market approach. Costs continued to soar. The system does not seem to respond to any economic stimulus.

The complexity of health care economics is further increased by the fact that, in health care, the patient rarely pays his own bill. In the past, increased costs were just passed on to the insurance companies who in turn passed them on to the employers who bought their employees' insurance. After the first few years of the DRGs, when the hospitals could not get enough money from the government prices to cover their costs, the hospitals started a practice of shifting costs. Medicare losses were simply passed on as higher costs for insurance companies. At this point, the insurance companies and the employers that pay them said, "We're not doing this any more." The largest insurance companies are demanding deep discounts from hospitals for sending their patients there. The hospitals are in a real squeeze for money to run the organizations. However, they have not totally run out of ways around the system yet, because they are still in business and some are still making profits.

It is very important that nurse administrators understand, not just the details of their budgets, but some of the values behind them. MacPherson (1989) wrote that, as leaders of the nursing profession are developing an ethic of a caring, health care delivery systems are moving toward increased competition and care-avoidance incentives. Certainly problems will arise as nursing attempts to implement a caring ethic when it runs into a wall of constraints that has been constructed by an economics-oriented health care system.

Ray (1989) said that bureaucratic caring can be unifying rather than alienating. If the whole system can understand and support a caring mission, even tough business decisions can be made with caring in mind. She suggests that health care organizations use cost-benefit analysis when deciding how to spend their funds. That process compares the cost of a program with its benefits. The problem with this method comes if the only benefits considered are economic. First, there are tangible benefits of some services that result in less use of health care. This is not always a benefit to the health care organization, who remains in business by continued health care services. Still, cost-benefit ratios need to be ascribed to new or continued programs. In addition, Ray insists that there are intangible benefits that should also be considered. Intangibles include avoidance of early death, pain, grief, or discomfort. So, when cost-benefit ratios are determined, they should include tangible and intangible health care benefits. In the past, failure to evaluate the benefits have worked against nurses who deliver care that increases the intangible health care benefits to patients. Ray said that nurses should be fully included in economic evaluations and should not let the intangible benefits be ignored.

Mark and Smith (1987) wrote about economics for nursing. In discussing budget and cost control, they advocate that:

> Above all, the nursing administrator must ensure that it is not staff nurses who are setting productivity, cost control, or quality goals. The managerial challenge is to motivate and direct nurses toward higher levels of performance. . . . Health care managers are responsible for directing employees toward higher levels of financial performance despite less favorable conditions. Although a health care organization may require higher quality and lower cost services, this does not necessarily imply they will have the resources to reward nurses who achieve exemplary performance.
>
> (pp. 262–263)

These are harsh words to the ears of nurses who want more than anything to implement caring. It sounds like we will not have enough resources to provide any kind of care at all. My own feeling is that, if you approach the heath care costs problems in that kind of a harsh way, you do not understand caring for yourself or others. I am not unaware that it will be a real struggle to find a balance between economics and caring, but it my impression that it will happen most successfully if we do the opposite of what Mark and Smith suggest. It is not a time to pull in the bureaucratic reins and crack the whip. It is the time to engage the nurses and other hospital employees to become a part of figuring out how to survive with our mission—caring—intact. When budgets got tight where I worked, the unit that had the greatest success was the one where the head nurse had said to the staff, "Here's what we have; how do we use it without losing our goals?" Certainly I have grave fear about how we are going to get resources for caring, but I do not think the American people will put up without it for long. Cleland (1990) wrote about the difference between needs and wants in health care. Patients may want things that the health care providers do not think they need. On the other hand, doctors may feel that patients need more than they want. Cleland wrote that society may or may not be willing or able to purchase everything that the provider may have identified as part of appropriate nursing interventions.

Cleland says that we need to use cost-effectiveness analysis and cost benefit analysis to help make choices in health care services.

Hailstones (1984) discussed the economic liberalism of the nine-
teenth and twentieth century when free trade, self-interest, private property, competition, and laissez-faire government were at their peak.
However, self-interest promoted greed, materialism, and abuse of economic liberty. Competition was inadequate to regulate abuses. Large
firms destroyed small firms, monopolies arose, markets were controlled,
and consumers exploited. Competition beat down wages to where the
market wage was less than the living wage. People were no longer able to
pursue the American dream. Governmental intervention was needed to
help even out the economy, and thus government regulated the railroads,
interstate commerce, antitrust, labor, public utilities, food and drugs,
social security, unemployment compensation, minimum wage, and fair
employment. The subsidiary role of the government causes the higher
units in the economy to give assistance to the lower units. The proper role
of the government in economic systems is to provide needed goods and
services that the capitalistic system will not. For example, there would
likely be no defense system under a competitive system since there would
be no way to make the venture profitable. Likewise, there are many
research problems that would go unaddressed (for example, orphan drug
studies) without governmental programs. Hailstones said that the goals
for the government economically are: 1. full employment; 2. stable prices;
3. economic growth; and 4. equilibrium in international trade. He stated
that the disadvantages of a market economy are:

1. recurring recessions;

2. presence of unemployment and poverty;

3. administered pricing by monopolists;

4. wasteful use of resources; and

5. unequal distribution of property and income.

Hailstones also reminds us that there are many gray areas in economics. After obtaining facts, establishing our principles, and drawing economic conclusions, we have to put them back in relation to our cultural,
social, political, and moral aspects of society. The difficulty in this is that
our values shift all of the time. Some of our societal values affecting health
care and their shifts in the past ten years include:

1. *Supremacy of life.* In the past, Americans have always placed great importance on life. In the health care business, that meant that when someone became ill, we were expected to do anything and everything to keep the patient alive. We used every means at our disposal to keep patients alive. Now we have Dr. Kevorkian who has created a national crisis because he helps patients die. And there are now debates about whether we can afford to spend billions of dollars on just keeping every patient alive. There is talk of rationing health care and perhaps not "going all out" for the terminally ill or premature babies who have a slim change of a quality life even if they can be kept alive with all of our technology. Many people have no desire to be kept alive if their quality of life is not good. People of all ages are preparing "living wills" that instruct the health care provider as to how much heroics they want done if they become comatose. The courts have upheld a person's right to refuse all medical treatment if they become totally incapable of living a meaningful life. So the value of supremacy of life—while still strong—is being challenged today, and heath care must find its own meaning for caring for patients that we once would never have questioned. This value, as many others, has a great deal to do with caring. A strong part of caring is relating with a person so closely that you perceive their reality. If that reality is not acceptable to the patient, then do we have a right to force them to live? What is the caring thing to do? This value also has a lot to do with economics—another collision between economics and caring unless we can find new ways to meet both needs.

2. *Rights vs. privileges.* There has been an ongoing values debate for years about whether health care is a right or a privilege. Few people would come out and say, "You can't get health care unless you can afford to pay for it." But our inattention to people without health care insurance has sounded that message loudly and clearly. The debate is more open now, with lots of press being given to the sick poor. Before I finish this book, I hope this debate has been settled and that every American has health care. What that will say is that health care is a right, not a privilege. The value of rights vs. privileges is in flux, but it has shaped our system for many years. Although unspoken, we are running the system as if health care was

a privilege. That has been very hard for nurses who have believed for many years that health care was a right. Perhaps this debate will be put to rest soon, but I have a suspicion that we have not seen the last of this values debate.

3. *Need vs. demand.* This is another value that has had a profound effect on health care. In years past, a patient got whatever the doctor said he/she needed. Then in the 1980s—when we were trying to make health care competitive—the patient got whatever they demanded. Right now the decision-maker seems to be the insurance carrier. They have put in utilization reviewers who, from their offices and having never seen the patient, seem to have the power to tell the patient's doctor, the nurse, and the hospital when to send patients home and what services they can get at home. With the possibility of new governmental health care reform, it is hard to say who will decide needs and demands. I just hope the system evolves to the point where the patient, health care providers, and government agencies cooperate so that the patient ultimately gets the care that helps them to a place of healing.

4. *Insurance mentality.* The idea for health care insurance began in the early 1900s. It was initiated by unions in big companies like the steel mills and railroads. The idea behind insurance was that a large number of people would pay into a pool of money that could be used by the few who got sick. We have initiated many kinds of insurances: life insurance, disability insurance, dental insurance, and health insurance, to name a few. Since the beginning, health care was a priority, since one major illness could be so expensive that it could wipe out the finances for a family. In other words, the many paid a little so that the few would not have to pay a lot for health care. For many years, people have felt protected because of insurance. But there have always been some people who could not afford it. In the past ten years, it seems like more and more people have lost their insurance, often when they lost their jobs. In addition, insurance companies have started calculating the insurance premium based on the person's health. Therefore, people who have a chronic disease cannot get health insurance from anyone. More and more, insurance has become something for the privileged instead of the many. This can be attributed in part to the

A Caring Approach in Nursing Administration

trend in this country to watch out for number one—ME! Altruistic values of volunteering and giving to others has diminished as the greed and sense of entitlement has grown for the above-average-income person. This change in basic values is not surprising when we think of American economic systems. America was founded as the land of the free, and our values are topped by the one that gets me the most. Bellah (1986) wrote *Habits of the Heart,* in which he analyzed American values during our history. He found that the number-one value is that of "rugged individualism." People came to this country to make better lives. Many were escaping religious or political persecution, and their greatest desire was to live their lives in freedom. This has certainly made our country strong and most people have prospered. But we have often turned away when people need help (especially long-term help). Bellah believes that if we do not rekindle some values about helping people in need, our civilization is on dangerous ground. I believe that the loss of the insurance mentality has had a divisive effect in our country, and that if we can re-create a successful insurance mentality, it can be a healthy step to a more compassionate America.

5. *Altruism vs. leisure.* This value structure relates closely with the last one, and is related to the dilemma of helping ourselves and helping others. Americans value money above most else, as money is our symbol of success. We will do most anything to get money. But about ten years ago, this value also changed. We had come to value our time as much as our money. Many people had "had it" with the gruesome work schedules, and some were even willing to cut back on money to have more free time. Then, in the past few years, working all hours has again become an organizational norm. This seems to be a schizophrenic value. Many Americans even spend their free time on competitive activities rather than relaxing or doing something to help another. One big way that this has impacted health care is that people no longer are as willing to give money or time to health care charities. That makes costs higher, because the patient pays for things that used to be donated. It also affects the work force in health care institutions. When working becomes a burden, nurses do not want to work double shifts, and many want

part-time work instead of full-time (which is no problem if handled properly). This is a value that affects health care either way it goes. If people are in a cycle of working long hours, we see more stress illnesses. If we focus on leisure time, there seem to be less inclination to donate time or money. Thus, health care costs increase and less funds are available.

6. *Litigation.* The increase in lawsuits has had a huge impact on health care. Not only are health care dollars channeled to lawyers and some to very deserving patients, but the fear of lawsuits has also had the effect of creating "defensive medicine." The insurance companies began to see increased numbers of lawsuits, and the amount of damage in health-care-related cases created a panic. Not only did their insurance premiums go sky high, but doctors also started to think of protecting themselves from suits. They ordered many more tests than were necessary and treatments that were of questionable value so that their patients would think that everything possible was being done. There are movements now to limit malpractice claims and the amounts of damages awarded. This may cause a lot of movement in the value concerning litigation.

7. *Feminism.* The values of feminism have had a great impact on health care as well. As more women have entered the workplace, their needs and opinions have become more insistent. In the past, women's work was so undervalued that nurses had little recourse but to accept the domination of mostly male administrators and physicians. But as women in the workplace began to assert themselves, so have nurses. Some nurses want to be associated with feminism and some do not, but I believe that feminism has had a positive effect on nursing.

One issue that is very difficult to figure out in nursing economics is nurses' wage and salaries. Even with all the feminism, women still make only about 69 percent of the wages of men in comparable jobs. Some women have been able to gain a lot economically, but groups of women, like nurses, have had a hard time trying to get improved compensation. During the late 1980s nurses were able to gain economically. There were nursing shortages, and hospitals were sometimes bidding for nurses by improving their compensation packages. With differentials, staff nurses were able to make $50,000 or more annually in some places. Benefits

A Caring Approach in Nursing Administration

such as child care, flexible scheduling, and decent pensions improved the overall compensation package.

Cleland (1990) wrote about wage and salary issues for nurses. She suggests that nurses get involved in job analysis and determining wage levels. I personally was involved in a hospital-wide job analysis program. In these programs, all jobs in the institution are graded on certain factors. A job score is then calculated based on work activities, stress, supervision, decision making, use of technical equipment, work schedules, work environment, social factors, and personal requirements. In our study, nursing came out very highly rated because of the knowledge needed, decision-making expectations, amount of supervision, and amount of responsibility for direct patient care. The one area that hurt nurses a lot was educational requirements. In the job analysis, we outscored pharmacists, physical therapists, and many others, but we were definitely hurt by the fact that nursing does not require a bachelor's degree. In the end, the job analysis was never implemented because it was too controversial, especially when it came to nursing. It was felt that if nurses' salaries were adjusted up to the level of the job analysis, there would be outcries from the other professionals in the organization.

The other way nurses' wages are determined is by market comparisons. This is a very frustrating thing, because the fact that wages have been depressed perpetuates itself when only market comparisons are used. Although the law is not supposed to allow businesses to meet and share wage information for the purpose of wage-fixing, it goes on all the time. When there are nurse shortages, hospitals may increase wages. But after the shortages are over, wages stabilize among organizations. Hospitals pay what other hospitals pay, regardless of antitrust laws.

Another problem in nursing compensation is wage compression—having very little difference in the bottom and top wages in a job classification. In nursing, it has not been uncommon to have less than 50 percent difference from the top to the bottom salary for staff nurses. Then there has been the problem of what to pay nurse managers. Cleland suggested a salary model in which there would be a difference of over 200 percent between grades of nurses. This is far from realistic. Longevity and differential compensation would be additional. She also wrote about the substitution of equipment for human effort. She says that it makes sense to replace workers with machines whenever the difference is

20 percent savings or more. I think there is some equipment that has saved on nursing hours, but in more instances than not, our new equipment causes more work, not less. Nevertheless, Cleland recommends four areas in which employment productivity may be improved:

1. Substitution of equipment for human effort.

2. Improved methods of work (for example, decentralization of decision making, primary nursing, some forms of case management, substitution of home care instead of hospitalized care).

3. Removal of unproductive practices (old policies or procedures, governmental and regulatory requirements).

4. Improved management of human resources (most cost-effective case mix of staff, retention programs, use of nurse specialists).

Cleland adds that, ultimately, increases in productivity are a justification for increases in compensation that exceed inflation rates. This rarely happens, however.

How do issues of wage and salary equate to caring? First of all, a nurse who is unhappy about her payment is a nurse who has a hard time being caring. If your work does not seem valuable enough for the organization to pay you well, it affects your enthusiasm for your work. Hertzberg found that wages are a primary dissatisfier for employees. They are not satisfiers—they do not make an employee happy if there are other problems—but they are an important determinate of a sense of worth on the job. Good wages also mean employees can take care of business instead of worrying about where their next meal is coming from.

Benner and Wrubel (1989) say that it is important for organizations to enable highly motivated and dedicated workers to perform at the level they want to perform. They iterate that nurses become very frustrated when the organizational environment does not permit them to deliver the best care.

> The consequences of delivering inadequate care due to work overload erodes the nurse's self esteem and causes real anguish. Although the nurse may be effective in performing the tasks of skilled nursing, she or he may not be able to be engaged in *caring* for the patient. . . . Knowledge is dangerous if it is divorced from caring, and that human existence is based on care. Caring and

A Caring Approach in Nursing Administration

caring practices must set the health care agenda and managerial strategies must be shaped to serve caring.

(pp. 384 and 400).

So, economics cannot be allowed to overshadow the goal of caring. That does not absolve nurses from being active participants in cost-cutting programs; it does mean that we must find ways to simultaneously attend to cost and caring. This is part of our professional responsibility.

Cleland (1990) wrote about the struggle over whether nurses are professionals. If we expect them to have a big impact on the future economics in health care, we must make them part of the debate. Nurses have a unique perspective from which to address health care economics. They are professionals with an interest in seeing their organizations continue to provide caring health care. In the debate over whether nurses are professionals, we are really asking who the nurse works for. Are they professionals whose main allegiance is to patients or employees whose allegiance is to the organization? Fortunately, they are a bit of both. Nurses will always put patients first, but because of our history, nurses have learned a lot more about how to "get around" within an organization for the sake of patient care. Nurses can bring a reality to business systems so they can remain fiscally sound without losing the mission of caring. As health care continues to evolve, nurses will need to be prepared to play a more active role in economics. They will need to act more autonomously in managing patient care and more cooperatively in fiscal affairs. Nurses can become "professnocrats"—a blending of the qualities of professional and bureaucrat—an expert in caring and an expert in organizational operations (Nyberg, 1991).

What can nurses do financially?

1. Become economically literate.

2. Design their own systems that are quantitatively and qualitatively sound.

3. Gather and keep good information about how patients felt about their care and how it could be improved.

4. Continue to personalize care and teach others in the organization to appreciate a caring approach.

5. Do not concede the control of finance to anyone outside of nursing—being your own expert financial consultant keeps this very important facet of administration in your control.

6. Be aggressive about creating new jobs for nurses; do not wait for someone to tell you how: assume you know.

7. Articulate caring as an ethically responsible economic possibility for health care organizations.

Nurses have major responsibilities in the financial arena in the future. We must change how nurses view themselves in relation to the system. They must see themselves, not as cogs in a bureaucratic machine, but as human agents in a very important system. We must remember that we have financial responsibilities to patients to improve their health with minimal costs. In the past, we worked on the premise that if a service had any hope of helping a patient, we got it ordered. In the future, we will need to ask ourselves the hard question, "What can I get for this patient that will impact his condition within economic realities?" We must change nursing from an eight-hour work shift to a caring responsibility for the whole patient. New systems can be implemented that can enhance patient care without raising costs. For example, case management, if used properly, can be a wonderful opportunity to demonstrate caring. It is an opportunity to stick with a patient throughout their illness and an opportunity to experience many transpersonal caring moments. As we develop more caring systems, the result may well be more cost efficiency as we develop deep understanding of each patient's needs. We can refine what services are offered and make patients feel like their every need was met. Caring and economics *can* be one goal, not two.

When I was working on my Ph.D., I concentrated on economics and human caring. I developed a theoretical framework to visualize how these two concepts could be addressed (Nyberg, 1990). In my first model (Model 7.1), I tried to illuminate the dichotomies involved in nursing administration. First, I showed the two types of philosophic thought: 1. physical/scientific, and 2. perceptual/humanistic. At the time I was writing, there was a lot in the nursing literature about these two ways of thinking. We perceived them as dichotomous. The model then showed the theory level that was identified as organizational theory and nursing theory. Again, these were presented as opposing theories. At the conceptual level, human caring and economics were the divergent views. By the time I

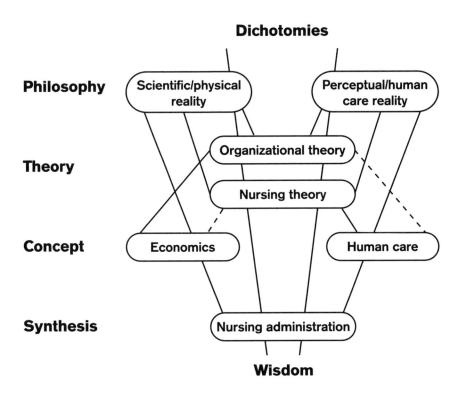

Dichotomies

Philosophy

Theory

Concept

Synthesis

Scientific/physical reality

Perceptual/human care reality

Organizational theory

Nursing theory

Economics

Human care

Nursing administration

Wisdom

MODEL 7.1

finished my work, it was clear to me that just presenting the problems of the dichotomies gave little help to practicing nurse administrators. In the revised model (Model 7.2), I showed the concepts of economics and human care as interdependent, and I showed nursing administration as nestled within nursing practice.

At this point in my thinking, I feel much more strongly about the overuse of dichotomies, which generally lead to more confusion than help. People do not look at the world as only scientific or humanistic; they do not study just organizational theory or nursing theory. We have seen in this chapter that caring and economics cannot be divorced from one another. We must learn to look beyond dichotomies to see how things are connected and interdependent. Jones and Alexander (1993) wrote about technology and caring. They are another two concepts that are viewed as dichotomous. Technology is seen as mechanistic, and caring as humanistic.

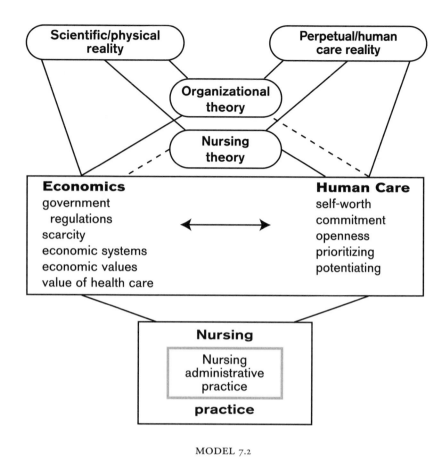

MODEL 7.2

Jones and Alexander argue that technology can have a more humanistic side. They write about technology as "hardware and software." The hardware side of technology is made up of machines and science. The humanistic, software side of technology is action performed from one to another, with or without tools or mechanical devices, to bring about some change in the recipient of care. They see caring and technology as two separate yet interrelated concepts that, when considered simultaneously, can be thought of as a unified concept—the "technology of caring."

We have a right to be very concerned about how caring can survive in the increasingly economically motivated health care system. But, rather than focusing on how different things are and feeling frustrated, we must take a proactive approach to our problems. One of the things that make me most hopeful about nursing's future is the high level of competency of the majority of nursing administrators. I feel confident that we *will* find interrelated concepts and ways to maintain and even enhance systems that allow nursing practice to be caring.

References

Bellah, R. N. (1985). *Habits of the Heart: Individualism and Commitment in American Life*. New York: Perennial Library, Harper and Row.

Benner, P. and J. Wrubel (1989). *The Primacy of Caring: Stress and Coping in Health and Illness*. Menlo Park, CA: Addison-Wesley Publishing Company.

Cleland, V. S. (1990). *The Economics of Nursing*. Norwalk, CT: Appleton and Lange.

Foster, R. (1987). Welfare economics and market failure. (unpublished).

Hailstones, T. J. (1984). *Basic Economics*. Cincinnati: South-Western Publishing Co.

Jones, C. B. and J. W. Alexander (1993). The technology of caring: A synthesis of technology and caring for nursing administration. *Nursing Administration Quarterly* 17 (2): 11–20.

MacPherson, K. L. (1989). A new perspective on nursing and caring in a corporate context. *Advances In Nursing Sciences* 11 (4): 32–39.

Mark, B. A. and H. L. Smith (1987). *Essentials of Finance in Nursing*. Rockville, MD: Aspen Publishers.

Nyberg, J. (1991). The nurse as professnocrat. *Nursing Economics* 9 (4): 244–247.

———. (1990). Theoretic explorations of human care and economics: Foundations of nursing administration practice. *Advances in Nursing Sciences* (1): 74–84.

Ray, M. A. (1989). The theory of bureaucratic caring for nursing practice in the organizational culture. *Nursing Administration Quarterly* 13 (2): 31–42.

Russell, L. B. (1986). Balancing cost and quality: Methods of evaluation. *Bulletin of the New York Academy of Medicine* 52 (1): 55–60.

Schroeder, C. (1993). Nursing's response to the crisis of access, costs, and quality in healthcare. *Advances in Nursing Sciences* 16 (1): 1–20.

Thaker, H. H. (1983). *Wage Setting and Evaluation: Economic Principles for Registered Nurses*. Kansas City: American Nurses Association.

CHAPTER EIGHT

The Search for Values and Ethics

In this chapter, we will explore the origins and perceptions of different ways of thinking about values and ethics. It is an important chapter because caring requires certain ways of thinking that are not always dominant in our society. Some of the material is organized around male and female characteristics. Let me say at the outset that I do not believe that all women think one way and men another. I do agree with many authors however, that you can define values and ethics that will be—the majority of the time—consistent with two ways of thinking about the world. If we use the words "caring" and "logical" as examples of values, it is probable that more females would relate to caring and more men would relate to logic. However, I certainly have met men who are very caring and women who are very logical. I also believe that these stereotypes are quickly breaking down and that men and women of the 1990s are working hard to communicate in one voice—a combination of caring and logic. For the sake of historical underpinnings, we will discuss the differences in men and women as described by several authors to see if there are underpinnings for our central concern—caring.

We start this discussion by examining Carol Gilligan's 1982 work, *In a Different Voice*. In the book, Gilligan traces the differences between the development of personality and morality of boys and girls. When a girl is developing her values in life, the basis of that development is a sense of sameness with their mother; thus the value of connectedness and relationships becomes very important in quite young girls. Boys, on the other hand, are treated by their mothers as different, and thus they spend their childhood focused on the value of separation. Boys play competitive games with clear rules and clear winners. Girls play games that focus on relationships and equality.

Gilligan states that in the history of psychology, and in life in general, most of the focus on success is measured by male goals of achievement. Authors such as Erickson, Piagett, Freud, McCellend, and Kohlberg used males almost exclusively when they developed theories of psychology and development. Thus, the model of success was the logical, competing, winning man. While women have taken care of men, that caring has not been valued in our society. The women's preoccupation with relationships was seen as immature and unimportant. Psychologists tended to see male behavior as the "norm," and female behavior as some kind of deviation from the norm.

Because of the differences in childhood, men and women tend to develop different fears. For males, the fear is of intimacy; for the females, the fear is of separation. Thus, men put their energy into succeeding in the business world and women hold the family together when it comes to relationships. The man will fear too much closeness in relationships and the women may fear too much success outside the home (worrying that the relationships may not be attended to properly). The men will have trouble admitting failing at work, while the women are afraid to take a stand on issues for fear of disturbing a relationship.

These factors result in moral judgments being made very differently by men and women. Men tend to want to apply rules to measure morality, while women want to take care of the people involved. Women's identity is defined in context of relationships and morality is a process of protecting relationships rather than balancing claims.

Gilligan does not see these differences as hopelessly incompatible. As men reach achievement, they may turn toward relationships; and as women achieve relationship balance, they may want to try the achievement side. Thus, though starting from very different points of ideology on justice and caring, men and women can come to a point of greater convergence in judgment and morality.

Gilligan's book is of enormous importance in nursing. It affirms the fact that, since women make up 95 percent of nurses, nurses tend to be very concerned about relationships. Since most doctors and health care administrators have traditionally been men, they focus on systems and the bottom line while nurses focus on the problems of taking care of patients—physically and relationally. With more woman becoming doctors and health care administrators, it will be interesting to see if things change. Nursing, devalued as women's work, may be given more credence in the future. In addition, younger people today have been raised with much less stereotyping, and it becomes unlikely that such sex bias will continue. Boys are being encouraged to have friends and think of others, and girls are encouraged to develop skills of logic and achievements.

This book is beginning to focus our attention on caring, female values. It lays the groundwork for us to begin to understand that the history of women has had a profound impact on nursing. As many authors point out, there is very little in history, the arts, and literature that is the work of women. Yet great women lived and gave of themselves at those times. The recognition may not have been there, but the women were. Now we are beginning to appreciate women in the arts and as professors and organizational leaders. Perhaps the history of our times will include more of the work of women.

The reason I decided to include this rather feminist material is because I think it relates to nursing. I think that over many years nurses have contributed to society with very little recognition. I believe that women's work—including nursing—was devalued, and that if we do not understand that, we do not understand our history, our present, or our future. The only reason to get feminist about it is to help nurses understand that they have been a product of the past, but they can now make themselves what they want to be in the future. It also is very confirming to have new authors that recognize the worth of women and women's work. It can make us proud and help us to understand that our values (relationships, caring, empathy) are just as important as the male values of logic, competition, and winning. I believe we need a world where people understand the two different kind of values and that we understand that one is as important as the next. In our ideal society, every girl and boy should learn about both types of values and try to assimilate them into themselves.

A Caring Approach in Nursing Administration

Now that we have learned something about value development in men and women, we can consider how the application of those values in our workplace (nearly half of the employees are women) is likely to be affected in organizations.

Sally Helgesen (1990) wrote a book *The Female Advantage: Women's Ways of Leading*. This author also points out the slow recognition of women's values in society. In particular, she takes issue with Mintzberg's famous study of the manager. She notes that even the term "manager" shows bias, and that Mintzberg included no women in his study of managers. Mintzberg reported on five managers and then wrote a description—a list, really—of what managers were like. Helgesen decided to do a study of female managers and contrast their characteristics with those of Mintzberg. Mintzberg found his male managers to be highly successful, powerful, controlling of information, decision makers, and good representatives for their companies, having authority and status. Words that depicted the male manager were: "contact," "decisional," "enterprise," "interruptions," "usurpation," "protection," "burden," and "shield." It was noted that men kept their work strictly separate from their personal lives. They identified themselves as who they were at work and generally spent little time at home. They felt pressured by unscheduled and conflicting demands, had a persistent sense of their own importance in the world, did seem to enjoy the texture of their days, took pleasure in accomplishing tasks, and saw work as a means to an end.

Helgesen's findings on female managers differed a great deal from Mintzberg's men. She identified their values as:

1. a willingness to look at how action will affect other people;

2. a concern for the wider needs of the community;

3. a disposition to draw on personal, private-sphere experience when dealing with the public realm;

4. appreciation of diversity; and

5. an outsider's impatience with rituals and symbols.

Rather than being upset at interruptions, the women seemed open to whatever contact they could get. Rather than hoarding information, the women saw their job as a "wheel" where information comes in and then is passed along to the right place. The women had a vision of society: they related their decisions to the effect they had on the role of the family, the

American education system, and even to world peace. They felt very strongly that they must make a contribution—not just to the company, but to the world. Where men harbored and bargained with information, one woman said she saw herself as a transmitter—picking up signals from everywhere and then beaming them out to where they needed to go. Words used to describe the women were: "flow," "interaction," "access," "conduit," "involvement," "network," and "reach."

Helgesen describes women's way of management as like a web. In the web, the figurehead is in the middle, not at the top. Authority comes from connection to people, not distance from below. In the web, the management's aspect of teaching is very important. The web is used to gain direct access to people and information and it allows the leader to test decisions on small parts of the web.

The other interesting part of Helgesen's book is that it talks about the difference between a leader having a vision or a voice. A vision is something that one person can have alone. It is visual—something that can be seen. It can be detached and objective. Most organizational texts talk about how important it is for the leader to have a strong vision. But Helgesen suggests that having a voice is more important. Having a voice means that you start with a vision, but that a voice is only a voice when someone is there to hear it. A voice starts with perceived truth, emerging from human circumstances where people listen and speak. The voice emerges from the interaction of people together. What is heard always influences what is said—speaking and listening suggest dialogue and interaction. Thus the leader develops a voice that emerges from her interactions with others. "Implicit in the use of voice as an instrument of leadership is the notion that care and empowerment are leadership tasks. Leading with a voice is only possible when one has reached a certain level of development as a person; otherwise the voice will not ring true" (pp. 226–230). Helgesen ends by pointing out how important women's ways of leadership are in the world today:

> Given the changing nature of both work and of people who work, there emerges a need for leadership who can stimulate employees to work with zest and spirit. . . . As women's leadership qualities come to play a more dominant role in the public sphere, their particular aptitudes for long-term negotiation, analytic listening, and creating an ambiance in which people work with zest and spirit

will help reconcile the split between the ideals of being efficient and being humane.

(1990, p. 235)

Helgesen's book gave me more hope for the future of organizations and their effect on the people in them. In particular, it offers great potential for caring values to be emphasized in management. Nurses' value to the organization increases as the values of women and caring take a more prominent place in society.

Another book of interest to nurse administrators is *Megatrends for Women* by Auburdene and Naisbitt (1992). It is a very upbeat book in which women's futures are clearly positive. They write of "critical mass" which, once reached, allows a process to become self-sustaining. They believe women have reached critical mass is many areas, such as politics, business, sports, fashion, and as social activists. Women's contributions in those areas will continue to be substantial. In other societal areas, women are increasingly active as well.

And so, it would seem, there is great need for women or people who use ethics and management principles like women. Woman bring new insights and methods that fit our time in organizational history. Once again, let us remind ourselves that it is not just physically created women that have all these leadership traits. Women's ways of leading constitute a paradigm, a new way of seeing organizations and leadership, and both men and women can enact these new methods. I know many men who lead as the women described and many women who would not understand a word of it. The point is not really one of sex—it's not who is better or worse—the point is that the female point of view has been overlooked and undervalued in organizations since their inception. Now we have newly identified ways of managing that females and males can value and use. It is a verification of women's worth and a step toward new ways of managing.

Nugent wrote in 1982 about managerial modes of thought. He postulated that there are two fundamentally different modes of thought—the rational and the intuitive. Rational thought emphasizes logic and step-by-step problem solving. It is the old management scientist approach. The intuitive manager, on the other hand, uses intuition, is globally oriented, pays attention to the gestalt of situations, relies on context, is relatively flexible, and needs less control over situations. Nugent does not relate these ways of thinking to men or women, but says that both type of managers exist. The real problem begins when the two types of managers try to work together. They frustrate each other with their different choices of management moves, and a power struggle can ensue. He suggests that managers sit down with each other and identify for themselves and each other which kind of managers they are. Then they can recognize each others' strengths and make a powerful management team.

Sargent (1983) wrote about androgynous managers. Traditionally, managers have been aggressive, rational, autonomous, and task-oriented. New managers need greater skill in dealing with people, expressing emotion, nurturing, supporting colleagues and subordinates, and promoting interactions. Sargent suggests androgyny, a blending of male and female characters that reside in varying degrees in each of us. She holds out the possibility that we might feel human and whole in the workplace and at home. Perhaps the competitive way of doing work can diminish and we will focus on collaboration and interdependence.

This is really what I dream of for leadership in the future. Caring and logic both have a place in health care, and blending them is ideal. I do think, however, that a time of emphasizing caring values must proceed the blending. It is impossible to blend things if only one-half of the recipe is valued. I think male managers need to be reading this type of material, but most might find it boring or bothersome. Since their way of managing has been dominant for so long, it is hard for them to see the need to change it. Perhaps only as the old ways of management fail, caring and female values will become more prominent in administration. Nurses can be there with caring values to pave the new ways of success for organizations.

Badarocco and Ellsworth (1989) wrote about a values-driven leader who strives to build an organization that is financially sound and a source of fulfillment and personal integrity to its employees. Some of the values they suggest are trust, fairness, respect for individuals, creativity and innovation, excellence, honesty, integrity, loyalty, humility, and serving others. Bracy, Rosenblum, Sanford, and Trublood (1990) wrote *Managing from the Heart*. They maintain that a company cannot maintain high-quality people, products, and profits unless it is managed with compassion and caring. Managers' jobs are to plan for, train, and motivate employees within the perspective of the company's mission. They believe that "managing from the heart" is how caring and respect can be spread throughout the business world.

A Caring Approach in Nursing Administration

So far in this chapter we have focused on values and caring and how a woman's approach to management can be helpful to an organization. We have studied how women manage differently and suggested that organizations of the future will need such management. We have recognized that women's ways of management do not necessarily belong to women, and we have heard how many authors believe all managers of the future will be more successful using a softer, more people-oriented approach in their organizations. We have inferred that values play a very large part in how people manage and are managed.

The question is, how does all this relate to nursing administrators? For me, it offers great hope. Nursing's values of relationships and caring are strongly emphasized. I believe that most nursing administrators will have the skills and the opportunity to influence health care organizations in very positive ways. If the nurse administrators are willing and able to articulate values and new ways of managing, they can lead the way to successful, caring health care organizations of the future.

The question then becomes, will added pressure on costs and efficiency allow space for values-driven management? Will the financial aspects take over? Will the system slip further back toward bureaucracy? Will health care executives be aware of these new ways of managing, or will they continue to want control and rule making. What will the tenor be of our new health care system? Will it become more people-oriented or devolve to treat people with little compassion because of a huge driving bureaucracy? Nurses can make a difference in all this. We are 3 million strong and have a better grasp of people-oriented systems than anyone. Will we speak up, stand up, and sit up with patients? Can we influence large organizations or perhaps start our own smaller ones where the new paradigm for management can be implemented for the sake of people— patients, employees, managers, doctors, and others? I think we can!

Now that we have discussed value systems for leaders and organizations, our attention will turn to look more closely at ethics and ethical systems.

Women's values and behaviors in an organization can change the ethics of how decisions are made. Ethics have also almost always been defined by men. Kohlberg's developmental level of ethics is one in which the person makes ethical decisions in dispassionate, distanced ways. Since women cannot seem to get over the "foolishness" of continuing to consider how ethical decisions affect people, they are ethically inferior as far as Kohlberg is concerned.

Ethics has become an important thing in our organizations, and our society. We do not want a president who is ethically weak, and we do not want to work for people who do not behave ethically. Marriner-Tomey (1988) defined nine different types of ethical positions:

1. "Utilitarianism"—do the greatest good.
2. "Egoism"—do what is best for oneself.
3. "Formalism"—be honest; remember the golden rule.
4. "Rule"—obedience to laws, rules, and professional codes.
5. "Fairness"—do what is fair for all involved.
6. "Priestly"—do what the highest power (God) edicts.
7. "Engineering"—decide ethics by presenting facts.
8. "Contractual"—identify general obligations.
9. "Collegial"—do what meets mutual goals.

(Marriner-Tomey 1988, p. 8)

These seem like reasonable ways to make decisions, but often they do not work. If we have two patients who need the same medicine and we only have one dose, how do we decide who gets it? Using utilitarianism, you may decide to give it to the person who can do the most good in society. If you use egoism and you are one of the patients, you take the drug yourself. Are there rules that decide this ethical dilemma? What is fair? What are all the facts, or do we have contract rules? Most nurses will solve this dilemma by moving heaven and earth to find a second dose!

Most health care organizations have formed ethics committees. But whose ethics are they using? The most common basis for ethics committees in health care is that of Beauchamp and Childress (1983). They say that ethical theories should be as clear as possible, and account for a whole range of moral experience. Their four ethical categories are:

1. Autonomy—decisions should be made by the individual involved.

2. Non-maleficence—do no harm.

3. Beneficence—do good.

4. Justice—do what is right for the group or society.

Again, a small example shows how hard it is to apply these categories. If Dr. Kevorkian has a patient who wants to die, how do we decide? Using the autonomy principle, we would let that patient decide for himself. Using the "do no harm" rule, we could not do anything to kill him. Using the "do good" rule is even tougher—who decides what is good? And justice—who decides what is just? Yet, these are the principles behind most medical ethics committees. Is there any doubt that nurses would have a very hard time sitting on such ethics committees? They are asked to decide the ethics of a situation without finding out who will be involved and whose interests are being served.

Cooper (1991) defined principle-oriented ethics and caring ethics. She wrote that a principle-oriented framework is the dominant conception of morality in this country. Principle-oriented ethics are characterized by their objectivity, strength of will, adherence to duty, and acting according to moral principles where everyone shares the same public norms, rules, and principles in a way that enhances moral predictability and consistency. In the ethics of caring, on the other hand, rules and principles play a secondary role in making moral choices. "Rather, moral concern is with needs and corresponding responsibility as they arise within a relationship" (p. 23).

Interdependence is valued in caring ethics as the ideal moral position. It reflects, not a helpless attachment, but an acknowledgment that individuals are naturally related to one another throughout life. Moral predictability and certainty are not goals in caring ethics, and the preferred moral response is individualization, guided by norms of friendship, love, and care rather than by abstract rights and principles. Cooper interviewed eight nurses and found that nurses relied on traditional moral principles (such as respect for persons, patient autonomy, beneficence, or fidelity) and at the same time relied on the moral response of care. As the nurse becomes engaged with the patient, tension develops between principle-oriented ethics and the moral response of care. The caring relationship provided the context for the nurse's engagement in the struggle and satisfaction of seeking meaning in the complex moral experience.

It should not come as a surprise that nurses use principle-oriented ethics since they are the basis of most ethics to which nurses have been exposed. What is interesting is that the nurses often find them to be lacking in being able to solve ethical dilemmas they deal with every day. The ethics of caring allows them to take each patient's individuality into account as ethics are determined.

Noddings' (1984) book *Caring* claims to describe a new ethic: a caring ethic. She does not approach ethics through law or principle or detached judgment. She defines a caring ethic that is "rooted in receptivity, relatedness, and responsiveness" (p. 2). It does not discount logic, but focuses rather on a longing for goodness. Noddings says that women are not without ethics, but when faced with a dilemma, they will often ask for more information. They want to see the person involved—to talk to them and see their eyes and facial expressions to receive what they are feeling. Noddings says: "Women can and do give reasons for their acts, but the reasons often point to feelings, needs, impressions, and a sense of personal ideal rather than to universal principles and their application" (p. 3). She rejects ethics of principle as ambiguous and unstable, as well as rejecting the notion of universality. In her description of caring ethics, each situation is its own world with its own variables and should be treated individually. To Noddings, ethics is coming to know another in such a way that an understanding develops about what is right in this situation for this person.

Caring ethics, as with all our other feminine material, is not isolated to women. But more women will want to face an ethical dilemma from a very personal point of view, which frustrates to no end the rule-oriented ethicist. Male nurses and many male doctors can also understand caring ethics. They can see the futility of applying principles that often conflict with each other and with the patient situation. They, too, want to know all they can about an ethical decision and then to make it in full partnership with the patient. Caring ethicists try to see situations as unique— one case only—and to understand that their responsibility is not to make decisions *for* the patient, but *with* the patient—with full knowledge of who the patient is and what his/her wishes are. Even in situations where the patient is comatose or a premature baby, the caring ethicist will immerse him/herself with the family and with the patient until what is right emerges from the situation rather than having it thrust upon them because of someone's list of principles.

Freel (1985) wrote about truth-telling in patient care situations. The issue is, "Should patients be told the truth?" This is a classic ethical dilemma. If the answer is yes, then which patient, what truth, who should be doing the telling? Is the nurse ever justified in deceiving a patient, not just by speaking an untruth but by silence, nonverbal pretense, or withholding of relevant knowledge? Since the patients' rights movement in the 1970s, professionals have been less likely to lie to patients. In the past, it was thought that the doctor should decide whether the patient should be told the truth, and he often didn't tell the patient the truth because it was

A Caring Approach in Nursing Administration

thought that the patient would "give up." Freel writes about the importance of veracity—the duty to tell the truth. He also points out that patients have a right not to know, if that is their wish. Not telling the truth may be right when the truth is impossible to know, the patient doesn't want to know, when the patient may be harmed by the truth, when it may be necessary to gain cooperation to facilitate a therapeutic situation, or when the patient may get confused. Mostly, though, nurses should tell the truth because: 1. it is essential to trust in the nurse/patient relationship; 2. patients have the right to know; 3. it is the moral thing to do; 4. it alleviates anxiety and suffering; 5. it is necessary to achieve patient/family cooperation; and 6. it meets the needs of the nurse and patient. There is the question of who decides whether or not to tell the patient the truth. In the past, it was clearly the physician, but now there is the thought that one profession should not have the right to tell another when to tell the truth. My feeling is that nurses can and should decide when to tell the patient the truth, but that it is best to discuss the issue with the physician so that agreement can be reached about talking to the patient. Sometimes the truth comes more appropriately from the nurse and sometimes it comes best from the physician.

It is very important that nurse administrators know and understand all kinds of ethics, but especially caring ethics. It allows them to sit back and trust that the nurse at the bedside is often in the best position to understand an ethical dilemma. The nurse administrator can help nurses explain their positions to administrators, doctors, etc., and validate the significance of this type of ethics. For the nurse administrator, again, what is good for nurses is often good for the administrator and the institution. Nurse administrators can use the caring ethic in all sorts of situations in their practice. It affects how they treat and support nurses, how they interact with other administrators and health care providers, and reminds them that the pulse of their job is caring in every situation.

Camunas (1994) did a nationwide survey of ethical dilemmas of nursing executives. They identified dilemmas over allocation of resources, access to care, and standards of care. There were conflicts about staff mix, numbers decisions, and staff reductions. Problems concerning individual patients were medical indigence, long-term care, prenatal care, and mental health. Patients in these categories frequently are not able to find care. There were conflicts about errors of staff, poor judgment, confidentially, veracity, and issues between superiors or subordinates. The nurse executives, though, were comfortable in making ethical decisions based on particulars of the situation, and did not require ethical formulas. Camunas suggests that education on ethics is needed for nurses at all levels in organizations. In the past, nurses acted from a goal-driven model (what the patient needed, he got), but in the future, a resource-driven model (what we have is what the patient gets) will prevail. Nurses will need to learn to use resources in the most efficient way as well as effective way to feel good about their work, or at least not encounter a severe disjunction between ideology and practice.

Ethics and values are among the most important issues for nurses today. The frustration about not being able to provide what they consider caring is very strong. We can discuss different systems, how to manage economically, and organizational models all we want, but the essence of any work is the ethics and values behind it, and they must be realized for caring to abound in our health care institutions of tomorrow.

In addition to patient care ethics, health care organizations are subject to *business ethics*. In the past, not much material was available on business ethics, and that which was available usually had categories, like medical ethics. Madsen and Shafritz (1990) say that business ethics are applied ethics—that you take theories and principles and apply them. Four ethical categories they recognize are: equity, rights, honesty, and exercising corporate power. Some ethical issues in businesses are: societal obligation, honesty, conflict of interest, employee rights, sexual harassment, confidentiality, and discrimination. These authors define two kinds of organizational ethics: "managerial mischief" and "moral mazes."

Managerial mischief includes illegal, unethical, or questionable practices of individual managers or organizations. The most common explanation of managerial mischief is that it is done by flawed characters with psychological dispositions that make them unable to control their desire to accumulate personal wealth. Another view is that their misconduct in business is a function of organizational pressures that push individuals into committing acts in which they would not normally engage.

I can understand both views, but I am most bothered by the view of organizational pressure. I think that is what is going on a lot in health care right now. I think managers are so acutely frightened about the potential of some health care organizations failing, that they are doing things that they wouldn't do. I think this is a very common reason for nursing's budgets

A Caring Approach in Nursing Administration

being cut to the point of reduced quality care. Managers are more concerned about their bottom line than about what the patients are getting in regard to quality and caring.

The moral mazes are far more subtle. Firms have obligations to suppliers, consumers, superiors, and employees. Sorting out the various obligations and responsibilities is not taught in business school. Examples of moral mazes are conflict of interest, employee rights, sexual harassment, propriety information, confidentially, and discrimination. So, business managers must deal with ethics in relation to the corporate mission, constituent relations, and policies and practices. They are often judged by whether they can bluff, withhold information, and "play the game," making ethics a lesser priority. To be a winner, it seems, a man must play to win. This gets us back to values and ethics. The ethics in business are still male-oriented. Maybe businesses will awaken to ethics that can be more caring as female managers take places in organizations.

I am sure each of you readers could come up with many examples of problems with business ethics. One that comes to mind is, "Should an operating room nurses let suppliers send them to a conference where they are submitted to many sales pitches and offered all kinds of gifts?" For nurse administrators, business ethics can take on much greater importance. For example, in health care, physicians are buying portions of labs and x-ray facilities and then sending all their patients to those facilities. Hospitals have also purchased outpatient facilities, rehabilitation facilities, and home care businesses. In one instance that I know of, a hospital started operating a home care business, and it put several other home care businesses (including the county home care operation) out of business. I always wondered if it was ethical to refer all our patients to our own home care. We said that we would give the patients a choice, but they were certainly steered to our facility. The federal government is now trying to get physicians out of owning businesses they refer to, but physicians are still doing it at this time.

Another variable in determining underlying values in organizations is whether they are for-profit or not-for-profit in structure. I have a basic instinct that says that health care should not be a for-profit business, but I am not blind to the reality that more health care organizations are becoming for-profit. The for-profit contingent would have us believe that they are so much more efficient that they can provide quality care which is less expensive in spite of the profit taking. At one time, this may have been true, but I think the not-for-profit organizations have become equally efficient. Profit is money unavailable for services. As efficiency improves to the maximum, the next step is reducing services and technologies. I would like to see all moneys earned go into caring for people with no insurance and keeping staffing levels high enough to have caring supported.

My belief is more of a ethical one than an argument about who is cheaper. I believe that health care should be a basic right for all citizens, and as long as we have a competitive environment, I do not believe we will have health care for all Americans.

That is not to say that for-profits do not ever serve community interests or worry about quality care. I think that only those for-profits with these goals will survive in the long run. The main variable is the value and ethics of the organization, be it for-profit or not-for-profit. If the for-profit attends to the needs of the communities and keeps staffing at a level where caring can be sustained, it may be an outstanding organization.

Another organizational movement is the formation of huge health care conglomerates. This is not just happening in health care. Banks, entertainment, and utilities are some of the industries consolidating. They are able to achieve somewhat lower costs, but the flip side is that there is less choice in products for consumers. In our country, creating conglomerates is taking the country by storm. In my city, we have several large conglomerates in health care. Inside the conglomerates, managers are being laid off and clinical practices are being standardized. They have achieved some economies of scale, and are in a more powerful position to deal with third-party payers. They are setting up their own PPOs and HMOs, and some are buying up physician practices.

I think that the values of conglomerates can vary from penny-pinching to expansive systems, depending on the way that they deal with patient care and employees. One value of nursing and medicine is autonomy in practice, and the conglomerates may damage this value if they try to standardize care too much or treat employees (including physicians) as interchangeable parts rather than valued individuals.

In the cases of profit motive and conglomerates, their natural tendency is to discount the values of caring and individualization. However, the values are defined by each organizational unit, and there is no reason that altruism and caring cannot become reality in for-profits or conglomerates. The defining variable is the people in the organizations. When nurses work in these organizations, they may find their jobs a little harder or a lot more meaningful. Nurse administrators can find many opportunities to assert their caring values no matter the size or structure of the organization.

Decision making in these organizations can become quite difficult. The bureaucratic ladder is generally large and so it is difficult to make quick decisions or changes. Nurse administrators may have difficulty placing themselves in a position of power or influence, and they must have great expertise in business and economics. Even the nursing structure may be very complex, and the chief nurse executive may have such a large span of control that it is very difficult to stay in touch with the nurses and nursing care. The nurse executive must carefully devise nursing systems that allow contact with nurses in their busy schedules. It helps to have an active number of nursing leaders who can be trusted to deal with nursing ethics and issues. Having a shared nursing philosophy and value system helps to define objectives and caring nursing practice.

Smith (1995) wrote about marketing ethics. Since health care organizations have initiated marketing, it is important to consider the ethics of marketing. Smith says that marketing strategies are increasingly subject to public scrutiny and are being held to higher standards. In the past, the marketing ethic was "caveat emptor" or "within the law." If a marketing method was legal, it was ethical. Smith said that marketing was easier when the economy was expanding. Now there is more pressure to market aggressively, but satisfying customers has become more important than ever. "Today, consumers' interests are increasingly favored over products. Consumers can make more informed choices, and less capable consumers are offered special protection" (p. 85). Smith suggests that the current period could be called the "ethics era." He believes that the ethic of "consumer sovereignty" is now appropriate. The three criteria of consumer sovereignty are consumer capability, information, and choice. Smith says that, in consumer sovereignty, the consumers exercise informed choice, and that this approach is now favored in marketing.

It is encouraging to see that marketing is now considering a higher level of ethics in their practice, but the principle of consumer sovereignty is difficult in health care because consumers often do not have enough information, capability, or informed choice. While patients are being encouraged to take a more active role in their health care, more and more people are being insured by HMOs, which limit choice. It is a confusing time.

Nash (1993) wrote about business ethics by contrasting a profit-only, short-term thinking ethic a "covenantal ethic." She defines business ethics as the study of how personal moral norms apply to the activities and goals of commercial enterprise. The major problem in business ethics today is that most managers are operating from a survival ethic. Their major goal is profit at any price, and the manager's main interest is in his own "profit." This self-interest has a way of turning into self-centeredness, which in turn, muffles the conscience. If the manager's efforts are constantly turned toward profit, it is very difficult to notice that ethical lapses are occurring and significant. Nash believes that management's working for survival (profit) is a real problem in today's business world.

> By limiting one's sense of purpose to survival, one limits one's performance as a person or company. A self-directed ethos motivates not excellence and innovation, but the construction of artificial barriers between management and marketplace . . . Self-interest positively obstructs characteristics of managerial excellence.
>
> (p. 75)

One of the side effects of the self-interest attitude is that employees do not trust that management cares about them, and that makes it likely that they will work carelessly and neglectfully. Nash even questions the benefit of performance-based reward incentives, since they merely increase the likelihood of shortsighted, me-oriented employees. The ethical manager has a responsibility to see that less-quantifiable, relationship-enabling characteristics such as "ability to communicate" or "success at empowering others" are taken into account during hiring, training, and performance evaluations.

Nash advocates for what she calls covenantal ethics. The term reflects the idea that capitalism is essentially a voluntary social contract between the public and businesses to fulfill certain mutually beneficial obligations. The chief goal of business is the creation and delivery of value to the democratic marketplace, and the chief responsibility of the marketplace is to see that businesses receives a fair return for provision of that value. The covenantal ethic calls for a blending of profit motive and other-oriented values that create trust and cooperation between people.

An important priority for the covenantal manager is integrity. Nash identifies business integrity as honesty, reliability, fairness, and pragmatism.

She believes that integrity is economically healthy and morally sound. The four essential characteristics of the covenantal manager are: 1. ability to recognize and articulate the ethics of a problem; 2. the personal courage not to rationalize away bad ethics; 3. an innate respect for others (empathy, self-sacrifice, altruism); and 4. personal belief in the worth of ethical behavior. Nash says that, if you understand the basic concepts of business to be about relationships of mutual benefit and the creation of value, then it makes personal morals and making money more compatible. The first purpose of business is the welfare of others; the second is profit. Service is the key. Managers using the covenantal ethic are relationship-oriented and more aware of a long-term perspective. The strengths of the covenantal ethic are:

1. It is oriented on a social relationship rather than on individual interest, reflecting the fact that business activity is a social activity involving multiple relationships.

2. It is pragmatic in several ways (describes what is generally agreed to be good business practice).

3. It recognizes that a logical appeal to self-interest is insufficient to motivate maintenance of ethical values in the marketplace.

4. It gives courage. By moving beyond thinking about oneself, it opens up a manager's moral dialogue to consider more than the weighing of personal risk and reward.

(Nash 1993, pp. 115–116)

Covenantal ethics offsets the power of ego and insists that managers develop the emotional capacity to listen and respect others, stay in touch with employees and customers, invite dissent and innovation, share experiences, ask questions, and acknowledge mistakes and uncertainty. In covenantal ethics, profit-driven motivation is replaced by value creation motivation, and the pursuit of efficiency is secondary to a sense of service relationships. With this theory, managers are more likely to be able to sustain their personal ethical norms and yet still build business strength.

The reason for exploring Nash's theory of covenantal ethics in such detail is that it is very compatible with our understanding of a caring theory, and it offers an ethical answer to the dilemma of economics and caring. Businesses can be viewed positively (creation of value), and the market can be viewed as positive (providing a fair return for value-creation). It emphasizes interdependence instead of a constant struggle for money and power. This is the only business ethic that mentions "caring." It is consistent with the caring attributes of putting relationships before rules, seeing things from the other's perspective, being fair and open and trustworthy, responding to positive and negative feedback, encouraging the potential of others, and the provision of a supportive environment. Nash believes that ethics are becoming more important in business, yet it feels like ethics are being suppressed in health care. It is probably true that most health care administrators are inherently ethical, but the current survival mode of management is not accentuating covenantal or caring ethics in the very industry whose major service is caring. In my experience, the emphasis of management on cost containment has left many nurses feeling like they are hanging onto caring by their fingernails. As I read Nash's book, I wanted to send it to health care administrators (including nurse administrators) to give them a literary reference about the importance of caring and ethics. I could think of moral dilemmas in my nursing administration when this book would have helped me stand firm in my conviction of caring. Nash's book could be used by nurses and nursing administrators to remind their organizations that profit is secondary to service.

Ethics and values are very important considerations for nurse administrators. They want to do what is best for patients, but sometimes that is not what is best for the organization. This is where caring ethics can help. Caring should be the goal of all health care, so, what is most caring is usually most ethical. Ethics and values are the basis for caring in health care.

Blanchard and Peale (1988) wrote that ethical behavior is related to self-esteem. People who feel good about themselves have what it takes to stand outside pressure and do what is right rather than do what is merely expedient, popular, or lucrative. Ethical power consists of purpose, pride, patience, persistence, and perspective.

Curtin (1992) says that ethics is knowing what is right; integrity is doing what is right. Success is being able to look back on your life and not having to be ashamed. She also says that the bottom line is self-respect— no one can define it for you, no one can give it to you, but without it, nothing else much matters.

Nursing administrators have a lot of ethical issues in and out of their jobs. Having an ethical framework is not only good for business, it makes your life have more congruence. I propose that the ethic of choice for nursing administrators is that of caring.

References

Aburdene, P., and J. Naisbitt (1992). *Megatrends for Women.* New York: Villard Books.

Badarocco, J. L. and R. R. Ellsworth (1989). *Leadership and the Quest For Integrity.* Boston, MA: Harvard Business School Press.

Beauchamp, T. L. and J. F. Childress (1983). *The Principles of Biomedical Ethics.* New York: Oxford Press.

Belenky, M. F., B. M. Clinch, Goldberger, and J. M. Tarule (1986). *Women's Ways of Knowing: The Development of Self, Voice and Mind.* New York: Basic Books, Incorporated.

Blanchard, N. and V. Peale (1988). *The Power of Ethical Management.* New York: Fawcet Crest.

Bracey, H, J. Rosenblum, A. Sanford, and R. Trueblood (1990). *Managing From the Heart.* New York: Delcorte Press.

Camunas, C. (1994). Ethical dilemmas of nurse executives. *The Journal of Nursing Administration* 24 (9): 19–23.

Cooper, M. C. (1991). Principled-ethics and the ethic of care: A creative tension. *Advances in Nursing Science.* 14 (2): 22–31.

Curtin, L. (1992). When catering becomes pandering. *Nursing Management* 23 (12): 24–25.

Freel, M. I. (1985). Truth telling. In McCloskey and Grace, eds., *Current Issues in Nursing.* Boston: Blackwell Scientific Publications.

Gilligan, C. (1982). *In a Different Voice.* Cambridge, MA: Harvard University Press.

Helgesen, S. (1990). *The Female Advantage: Women's Ways of Leading.* New York: Doubleday Currency.

Madsen, P. and J. M. Shafritz, eds. (1990). *Essentials of Business Ethics.* New York: Meridian Books.

Marriner-Tomey, A. (1988). *A Guide to Nursing Management.* St. Louis: C.V. Mosby.

Nash, L. (1993). *Good Intentions Aside: A Manager's Guide to Resolving Ethical Problems.* Boston: Harvard Business School Press.

Noddings, N. (1984). *Caring: A Feminist Approach to Ethics and Moral Education.* Los Angeles: University of California Press.

Nugent, P. S. (1982). Management modes of thought. *The Journal of Nursing Administration* 14 (5): 19–25.

Ray, M. A. (1987). Health care economics and human care in nursing: Why the moral conflict must be resolved. *Family and Community Health* 10 (1): 35–43.

Sargent, A. G. (1983). *The Androgynous Manager: Blending Male and Female Styles for Today's Organization.* New York: American Management Association.

Smith, N. C. (1995). Marketing strategies for the ethics era. *Sloan Management Review* (Summer): 85–95.

Chapter Nine

Research and Caring

This chapter will address the topic of research in general and specifically as it relates to caring. The chapter will not be exhaustive of the material available on research—that would take another whole book, but it will discuss the two major types of research and then see how those methods have been used in research in general, nursing administration research, and research on caring.

Nursing research, according to Cronin (1993), is the pursuit of scientifically based knowledge on which the practice of nursing can be based. Hinshaw (1989) reminds us of the complexity of phenomena in nursing practice. Most of the questions that are raised are multivariate and often involve several levels of the health care system. That is, most nursing care outcomes are partially the result of care by others (such as doctors, physical therapists, and others), so it is difficult to study patient care problems and specify exactly what the results of nursing care are. Hinshaw says that questions to be considered when setting research priorities are: 1. how do the discipline's priorities fit within the major health needs of society? 2. how can research priorities be identified and operationalized professionally and organizationally while allowing for scientific creativity and guidance of the discipline's body? and 3. because of the number of high-priority areas of study, how can the major questions in each area be identified while still allowing the addition of new priorities as society and nursing change?

Polit and Hungler (1983) wrote a well-known classical text on nursing research. They wrote that the ultimate goal of any profession is to improve the practice of its members so that the services provided to its clientele will have the greatest impact. Development of a scientific body of knowledge can be instrumental in fostering a commitment and accountability to patients. These authors believe that a professional nurse should base as many decisions and actions as possible on scientifically documented knowledge and seek to find scientific answers to problems.

Polit and Hungler stress that much of the early research was focused on nursing education, and time and motion studies. In the 1960s, nurses began to identify conceptual frameworks that would be developed into the earliest nursing theories. In the 1970s, research focused on the preparation of nurses and some research about the improvement of client care. Then in the 1980s, the focus became primarily patient care outcomes. There were also many studies about different types of nursing care delivery systems.

Polit and Hungler are focused on the scientific problem-solving method. They define the scientific process as objective and based on hard data (data that can be seen, felt, etc.) that could be analyzed with mathematical manipulation. Their book was used as the best one available to teach research methods for a long time. But, in the late 1980s, discussion began about less "scientific" methods of studying nursing practice. It was a time when the major paradigm of science was being questioned because there were problems that science just did not answer. A movement began that called for more qualitative methods of research. Now, in the 1990s, there is a strong movement that calls for studies that examine the lived experience of nurses and patients. This movement has led to new research methods like phenomenology, grounded theory, ethnography, and case studies. This type of research assumes that the researcher is a part of the research, not an objective bystander. The goal is not to gather scientific data that can be mathematically manipulated, but rather to rigorously study a phenomena to find the meaning of situations and relationships that cannot be studied scientifically.

When Polit and Hungler say "scientific," they mean objectivity and mathematical oriented. Actually, the word "scientific" can be used to described the newer methods also. For example, Watson calls her preferred research "human science." Other disciplines also do research which is not scientifically based if you define scientific as objectivity and mathematically based. The new qualitative researchers are as interested in the discovery of new knowledge as the more traditional researchers. It is just that they believe that some knowledge can only be discovered by research methods that include the researcher in the process of learning. For example, trying to find out about how patients feel about their care can be done with a scientific questionnaire, but the data would probably be less rich and meaningful than if a qualitative study was done where patients could talk directly to the researcher. No matter how good one tries to make a questionnaire, some of patient's experience cannot be captured by it. Yet, a good discussion may reveal feelings that the researcher never even thought to include on the questionnaire. Qualitative research is a process. One comment may lead to the exploration of new ideas, and the researcher may learn just by watching the patient—he/she may look scared or happy or mad. Because the researcher is there interacting with the patient, new knowledge can be discovered.

Both types of research are useful in their own way. L.C. Dzurec (1993) wrote that quantitative methods are presumed to be the method of choice for empiricist research, but qualitative methods are appropriate for research conducted within the phenomenological paradigm. The empiricist paradigm focuses on a reality that can be understood by studying physical topics to determine cause and effect based on laws of nature. The phenomenological paradigm believes that there are realities in life that cannot be seen or measured. Reality includes feelings, perceptions, and intuitions. Researchers must think carefully about what they want to learn, and then decide which method will best fit the problem at hand. Some nurse researchers believe that these paradigms and their respective methods are mutually exclusive, but the literature is now reflecting an evolution toward integrative methods. Dzurec says that quantitative studies depend on assumptions of probability, and qualitative studies depend on description and inferences. But both methods make interpretive, narrative statements about the implications of their data. Both attempt to construct explanatory arguments from their data, and both recognize the integral nature of human beings and the environment. Dzurec defines science as the practice of adopting a prescribed set of methods and assumptions for all investigation. This definition would allow for quantitative and qualitative methods.

Watson (1985) discusses the difference in the traditional science paradigm and a human science paradigm. The traditional approach follows a research tradition that concentrates on issues such as objectivity, fact measurement of smaller and smaller parts, and issues such as instrument reliability and validity. Human science, however, encourages exploring the subjective part of life, which includes metaphysics, aesthetics, humanities, and art. The human-science approach utilizes studies that allow the researcher to be involved in the clinical research process rather than being distant, objectively remote, and primarily concerned with the product of science.

Some researchers use both qualitative and quantitative methods. They "put them together" by a process called "triangulation" which involves taking two known or visible points and using them to plot a third point. The purposes of doing this (according to Breitmayer and Knafl, 1994) are confirmation and completeness. Confirmation refers to selecting data collection instruments or techniques whose strengths and weaknesses are known and counterbalancing. The goal of completeness is to study varied dimensions of the area of interest to achieve coverage of different aspects of a phenomenon. Using two or more measurements can help one see more completely the item or situation to be studied. If this is done, however, the researchers must understand that they are not just using two measures, they are mixing two philosophies. They must be clear about what they are measuring and what each measure means to the understanding of the whole phenomenon.

Having discussed how researchers work, it is now important to discuss nursing administrators' responsibilities involving research. Hinshaw and Smeltzer (1987) say that to establish a successful research agenda in a practice setting requires a commitment to the value of research in guiding decision making and allocating and generating resources. The challenge is finding administrative and clinical problems that are researchable, and then balancing the practice setting's need for immediate information against the scientific need for longitudinal and replication studies to confirm research findings.

Smith (1993) wrote that nursing administrative research is the study of the health of the organization within the context of the social, political, and economic environment. The nursing administrator promotes healing, well-being, and health for patients and for the organization. Smith believes that nursing's metaparadigm focuses on human beings and that nursing administration should view their work as focusing on the organization as a living system of people with perceptions, feelings, and concerns. Nursing is more likely to view patient care as the reason for health care organizations, and they are most likely to argue the priority of quality and humane patient care and work environment. Nursing administrators can influence the other administrators in the organization to address the environment and express caring as a central concept. So, the nurse administrator should do his/her own research and encourage nurses throughout the organization to be involved in research. In addition to that, the nurse administrator must find the financial and supportive resources for research within the organization. It is increasingly difficult to find funding, but the actuality is, that if we do not do the research, there is a cost in terms of not finding new ways to do and organize nursing so that cost savings can be achieved.

The American Organization of Nurse Executives' report on nursing administration research defines nursing administration research as the "scientific inquiry of the factors that influence the effective and efficient organizational delivery of high-quality nursing services" (Hinshaw 1989, p. 251). This indicates that there is research that is unique to nursing administration. It involves developing models and systems that enhance nursing. The complexity of such problems makes it a very big challenge indeed. The American Organization of Nurse Executives identified four research categories: 1. practice and administrative systems; 2. support services; 3. documentation; and 4. education.

Schultz and Miller (1994) did a survey of nursing administration research in the 1980s. They wrote that nursing administration research has been slow to develop, partially because there has been confusion about nursing administration as a nursing specialty. But, since the pressures of major economic and regulatory changes, there has been increased acceptance of nursing administration as a practice within nursing that is crucial to the future of the nursing profession. Nursing administrative research usually includes looking at groups, units, or organizations as the units of analysis. It attempts to find systems improvements, overall improvement of nursing outcomes, and workplace issues. The kind of

A Caring Approach in Nursing Administration

nursing administration research reviewed by Schultz and Miller are resource utilization, costs of delivery of nursing, quality of nursing care and nursing processes, subcomponents, interaction, and social and technical work environments. They found through their literature review that the evidence clearly directs administrators from hierarchical structures and patriarchal management styles toward participative decentralized models. They found a disappointing disparity between cited research and the degree to which it has impacted organizational and health care delivery systems. There is substantial need for continued research focused on the health characteristics of persons served by nursing care organizations. They found a frequent lack of theoretical frameworks within which to ask research questions. We need to develop theoretical frameworks that are congruent with nursing's defining concepts and assumptions.

Sperhac, Haas, and O'Malley (1993) say that, in our cost- and quality-conscious health care environment, the value of nursing research is increasingly important. Their perception is that research is still not part of the work a day world. The challenge is to shape an environment where conducting and participating in nursing research can become a clinical practice norm. To that end, they devised a program to free up nurses for short periods so that they could initiate and complete a clinical research project. They started a sabbatical and scholar program where any nurse could propose a research project that could be funded up to $20,000 and six months' paid time. Their program has been very successful. They say that when nurses see the opportunity and support for conducting clinical nursing research, they come forward with well-formulated research questions. Because they are practicing clinicians, they know the issues and can quickly identify variables and obstacles. The most impressive sign of this program's success is that 99 percent of the nursing staff are aware of changes in nursing practice related to the sabbatical and scholar program. It is an example of how nursing administrators can encourage research and research-based practice for the nurses in their organizations.

Blegen and Goode (1994) wrote that one of the goals in nursing is to place nursing practice and administration on a strong foundation of knowledge supported by research. They are concerned, as I am, about the dissemination of research results so that the results can be applied to nursing practice. These authors were involved in a program to bring academic researchers together with practicing nurses to conduct meaningful research. They did studies of job satisfaction and nurse autonomy, and the results were that the nurses did indeed sense improved job satisfaction and a sense of autonomy. They felt that the academics and practitioners worked well to develop useful research with application to practice.

Another area of nursing administrative research is in the development of new patient care modalities or systems. Rizzo, Gilman, and Mersmann (1994) say that too often care delivery changes are put in place with inadequate planning and very little evaluation. They used a research approach to implement a change in their nursing organization. The study showed a savings of $30,000, while hours of nursing care increased only slightly (through the use of more LPNs and nurse-aides). There were no changes in quality of care measures, and care planning and discharge planning showed steady improvement.

It is a refreshing change to see administrative research used for making change in nursing systems. For a long time, most changes were made by taking a shot-in-the-dark implementation followed by finding success in areas where the administrators knew it would be. So, we can begin to see the efficacy of nursing administrative research. It is often difficult to find the time and money to do the studies, but not doing them may in the end be more expensive. For example, nursing seems to get caught up in fads such as team nursing, primary nursing, and now case management. If it works in one institution, it is assumed that it will work anywhere. It makes a lot more sense to set up a study in each site to see if the results are the same. I was involved in one institution where a new system was put in place. The results were disappointing, but the organization did not want to be seen as negative, so it did not publish the results of the study. I am afraid this happens all too often, and that gives us tainted information about new systems and ideas. Research is valuable no matter what it shows. In fact, negative results could be very helpful in keeping organizations from costly mistakes. Ideas or systems must be evaluated for each institution because each institution is unique. The ideal of nursing administration research is to improve planning, implementing, and evaluating innovative programs.

Another area that needs to be attended to is how organizational or extraneous variables affect clinical studies. Miller (1994) addresses that problem in her research work. She believes that "nurses have always been at the forefront of efforts to create health care systems that support positive outcomes for patients. However, few studies have been conducted on the relationship of nursing care delivery systems and patient outcomes" (p. 107). Miller's work is focused on the research of contextual variables. She defines context as a general setting or set of circumstances in which a particular event or situation occurs. She believes that many of the studies done about nursing care delivery have not taken into account the many organizational and environmental factors. For example, most studies do not attend to changes in the marketplace, changes in economic constraints, changes in political influences, changes in technology or procedures, changes in competencies, or changes in management or management philosophies. Nurses know that such variables can greatly affect the patient care intervention they may be studying, but no one has figured out how to measure the contextual variables involved. Miller and others are developing a tool to measure contextual variables. She believes that measures of outcomes should be considered along with the contextual variables. She says that combining the knowledge from clinical studies and outcomes research with systems analysis may provide the best data on the complex reality of patient care research. Miller writes that "to have significant impact on patient outcomes, it is important to have educators who are willing to teach flexibility and autonomy, researchers who are willing to try new designs and methods despite the flaws, administrators who are willing to create new systems that will improve the context of care for all concerned, and most of all, clinicians who are willing to practice differently and with the patient's interest paramount" (p. 114).

Another important avenue of nursing research is outcomes research. This type of research can be done by nurse administrators or clinicians, and it is definitely being given major attention in the current health care system. Brett (1989) brought attention to the need for outcome research in nursing. In the past, the usual outcomes were morbidity, mortality, and complications. Now, nursing is attempting to develop its own nursing care outcomes. Brooten and Naylor (1995) wrote that measuring patient outcomes dates back to Florence Nightingale, who used mortality and morbidity measures during the Crimean War. In 1962, Aydolotte examined such outcomes as number of days in bed; fever; doses of narcotics, analgesics or sedatives; mental attitude; skin color; and patient and doctors evaluation of nursing care.

Bower (1994) believes that outcome research is the best way to demonstrate nursing's place in changing systems and models in health care. She says: "A sole focus on cost without a consideration of quality, access, and continuity paves the way for decisions which are short-sighted solutions to complex questions. Nursing must make its point from research that demonstrates the important and desirable outcomes which are a direct result of nursing actions" (p. 4). Nursing has involved itself in many cost studies, and that cannot stop: as the system becomes more cost conscious, so must nursing. Nursing must be a willing participant in developing less-expensive systems, but I agree with Bower that we must continue to make our top priority quality of care. For many years, nursing did not base its practice on research, but in the last two decades, more and more nursing research has been done, and nursing's knowledge base is increasing at a faster and faster rate. Nursing research has become an accepted knowledgeable endeavor.

Hegyvary (1991) says that we must account for what we do, why we do it, what we produce, and what it costs. Outcome research must be a priority as we tie cost to quality in health care. Outcomes determine what conditions and actions produce what outcomes. Some outcomes in nursing are staff satisfaction, levels of staff performance, and costs per patient-day. These are nurse-related outcomes. However, the current thrust is for patient-related outcomes from nursing care. At the micro-level, one can examine individual patient responses to nursing care. At the macro-level, one could examine clinical services to groups or communities of people.

Waltz and Strickland (1988) measured nursing outcomes such as levels of stress of discharge, compliance, goal attainment, pain, risk, fears, coping behavior, and others. Shiber and Larson (1991) addressed the outcomes of the caring process such as nurturance, growth and development, competence for the patient, and the extent to which patients perceive that they have been cared for.

Bostrom and Wise (1994) believe that there is currently a nine- to fifteen-year gap between discovery of potential innovations and implementation. This is a very big problem because knowledge in nursing and technology is expanding every few years. Nursing needs to find ways of getting new knowledge into nursing practice as fast as possible. Bostrom and Wise advocate a computerized program (called RARIN) that allows nurses access to much of the nursing literature. This seems like a very good thing, but the RARIN system will only be valuable if it is used by nurses in all settings. In order for that to happen, nurse administrators must learn about the system and make it available in practice settings.

Smith (1993) said that, if we assert that there is distinct knowledge in nursing, it is incumbent on us to explain and support the contention through development of nursing theory and research. I agree with this premise also, but again the statement only counts if nurses everywhere know and use the theory and research. Most of the research reports are in scholarly journals, and practicing staff nurses are not likely to read them. So, knowledge is one issue and dissemination is another. Nursing administrators can have a big effect on the dissemination of nursing knowledge. They can use situations that let people know that the nursing administrator reads and incorporates new nursing knowledge. In addition, the nursing administrator can contribute to the literature and send appropriate articles to nurses in all parts of the organization to encourage them to be up-to-date.

Now that the importance of research in general, and to the nursing administrator in particular, has been discussed, our attention will turn to some of the research on caring. Caring has always been a priority in nursing, but it became a common research topic after Watson's 1979 book, which defined caring as a nursing theory. In 1986, an issue of *Topics in Clinical Nursing* reported several research studies on caring. In that issue, Wolf wrote about the creation of the Caring Behaviors Inventory (CBI) which was produced using a collection of caring words and phrases that the author felt may indicate caring in nurses' clinical practice. Nurses ranked seventy-five caring words and phrases and then the author selected the ten highest ranked ones. They were: "attentive listening," "comforting," "honesty," "patience," "responsibility," "providing information so that the patient or client can make informed decisions," "touch," "sensitivity," "respect," and "calling patient or client by name."

Swanson-Kauffman (1986) studied caring in the instance of unexpected early pregnancy loss. She interviewed twenty married women who miscarried prior to sixteen weeks gestation. She found the process of loss that followed miscarriage included: 1. coming to know; 2. losing and gaining; 3. sharing the loss; 4. going public; 5. getting through it; and 6. trying again. Caring was seen as knowing, being with, doing for, enabling, and maintaining belief. These attributes seem to be specific to her population.

Mayer (1986) studied cancer patient's and their family's perceptions of nurse caring behaviors. She found that the effects nurses have on patient's welfare is greatly influenced by their relationships. The caring process included: 1. attributes of the caregiver and receiver; 2. interpersonal process; and 3. behaviors that convey caring. She recognized the importance of activities requiring technical skills and competence, but also felt that more expressive activities should not be undervalued.

Brown (1986) studied caring from the patient's perspective. She interviewed fifty patients and found eight themes of care: 1. recognition of individual qualities and needs; 2. reassuring presence; 3. provision of information; 4. demonstration of professional knowledge and skill; 5. assistance with pain; 6. amount of time spent; 7. promotion of autonomy; and 8. surveillance. Brown wrote that it was fundamental to the experience of care that the patients have confidence in the ability of the nurse to provide the necessary physical care and treatments. Once competency is established, the more expressive caring activities become important.

Riemen (1986) did a phenomenological study to identify patients' descriptions of caring interactions with nurses. The surprise of this study was that the patients identified many noncaring incidents. Examples of noncaring were: being in a hurry, doing a job, being rough and belittling patients, not responding, and treating patients as objects. It seemed to be easier to say what caring was not than what is was. Not once was an ill-performed technical procedure mentioned. Rieman wrote that existential presence in a caring transaction does not have to involve extensive time; rather, in each interaction, the nurse must be truly present in thought, word, and deed.

Hutchison and Bahr (1991) studied caring among elderly nursing-home residents. They found that caring behaviors were a universally important means for residents to maintain their esteem, self-identity, and continuation of personhood. They identified the properties of caring as protecting, supporting, confirming, and transcending. The study was done using a grounded theory approach including interviews and observation. This was a very different population of patients, and the study shows the importance of caring to people of all ages.

On the other end of the spectrum, Swanson (1990) wrote about caring in a newborn intensive care unit (NICU). She used a phenomenological approach, which she says requires a researcher who has: 1. a question about a phenomenon; 2. the capability of intuiting the experience of those who actually live the experience; and 3. the rigorous plan for data gathering that is congruent with how the phenomenon might exhibit itself in reality. She concluded that there were four basic processes of nursing in the NICU: caring, attaching, management responsibility, and avoiding bad outcomes. Certainly, in an NICU, knowledge and skills are very important, and yet this study validated the importance of the interpersonal part of caring.

The studies just reviewed were predominately qualitative inquiries that examined caring between nurses and patients. They are an important contribution that has helped move caring from a conceptual ideal to a way of practicing nursing. Other studies followed that were more quantitative, and therefore more generalizable (larger groups of people can measure caring with a quantitative tool, so the results are more likely to be repeatable in other settings).

In 1987, Larson did a study of cancer patients and professional nurses' perceptions of caring behaviors. She developed a questionnaire (Care Q) that she administrated to nurses and patients. She found a strong difference in the groups of nurses and the group of patients. The nurses identified measures of comfort and trusting relationships as most important, while the patients identified monitors and follow-through as most important. This study really surprised me. We all assume that patients view caring as we do, yet this study did not indicate that fact. When I think of my own hospital experiences, I guess I would want technical knowledge first, but then supportive care would be important. If you did not have the technology, it might result in harm or maybe even death to the patient. But, if you do not have the comforting part of caring, hospitalization can be a lonely and sterile experience.

Mayer (1987) used Larson's Care Q tool to study nurses' and cancer patients' perceptions of caring behavior. She found a significant relationship between patients' and nurses' rankings for all fifty items, but there was no agreement on the five most important behaviors identified by nurses and patients. There was agreement, however, on three of the least important behaviors. Nurses ranked "listens to the patient" and patients ranked "knows how to give shots, IVs etc." as most important. This follow-up study confirmed the others using Larson's Care Q tool.

Ray (1987) did a study of technological caring in a critical care unit. She used an interview and observation approach and found that critical-care nurses displayed both technocratic aspects and the caring aspect of nursing. Though one may think of critical-care nurses more as technocrats than as caring, Ray found that the nurses used ethical and moral processes in their work. Expressions of human caring included maturation, technical competence, transpersonal caring, communication, and judgment. Ray found that when the nurses' needs were met in mastering the machinery, they could focus on meeting the patients' other needs. Burn out occurred when the nurse became overwhelmed by the equipment. There were sometimes conflicts of values between life and death. Initially, most patients were hooked up to lots of equipment, but the nurses seemed to sense when the patient was suffering and not being helped by the aggressive treatment. At that point, the nurse began to take action to protect the patient against aggressive treatment by communicating with the doctors, family, and peers. Ray concluded that critical-care nurses responded in caring fashion that arose from a sense of bonding or attachment to the patient. Again, we find the importance of technology, this time by nurses. But the study also confirmed the opinion that interpersonal caring is still important.

Ray (1989) also did a study about bureaucratic caring that has already been mentioned. In this study, she used a grounded theory approach to define how caring was enacted in an organization. She found that informants began by describing caring in humanistic terms, followed by terms related to the informant's role, and finally with respect to the informant's position within the organization. She concluded that bureaucratic caring is not only possible but necessary to the health of the organization and the patients it serves. This study broadened the concept outside of nursing. It found caring in unlikely places, but it helped me to understand that caring goes beyond nursing's boundaries. This study is an example of nursing administrative research even though the concept being studied is a clinical one.

Valentine (1989) also studied caring in an organizational setting. She found that the core of caring consists of psychological elements put into action in a context that is either social or physical in nature. Elements of caring included communication, teaching, comfort, touch, and administration of treatments. She concluded:

A Caring Approach in Nursing Administration

Caring is more than kindness. It is also the cognitive aspects of the nurse-patient relationship such as the knowledge the nurse brings to that relationship, the availability of the nurses, the performance of tests and procedures with skill and care, the honesty and integrity of the nurses, and the ability of the nurse to respect the individuality and autonomy of the patient. . . . Patients do not want nurses to sit with them and hold their hand; they do want them to be confident, friendly, and knowledgeable in their interactions with them.

(p. 33)

Again, there is the issue of the technical aspect of caring. As you recall, Watson wrote about the importance of technologic knowledge and skills in caring. She does not see them as exclusive from one another. She believes that caring requires technical competence as a part of care. I agree that caring encompasses knowledge and skills. I think that is what the patients in the early studies were trying to communicate.

Wolf et al. (1994) studied caring quantitatively, using the Caring Behaviors Inventory (CBI). They point out that caring is an example of nurses' hidden work that may go unrecognized by patients unless the behaviors and attitudes that constitute caring are missing. They define caring as "an interactive and intersubjective process that occurs during moments of shared vulnerability between nurse and patient, and that it is both self- and other-directed. Caring is directed toward the welfare of the patient and takes place when nurses respond to patients in a caring situation" (p. 107). They had 541 subjects in the study, which was done to validate the CBI tool. Using factor analysis, they defined five dimensions of caring: 1. respectful deference to the other; 2. assurance of human presence; 3. positive connectedness; 4. professional knowledge and skill; and 5. attentiveness to the other's experience. This description of caring is inclusive of skills and personal relationships.

Larson and Ferhetich (1993) studied caring in relation to patient satisfaction in hospitalized patients. They were using a revised version of the Care Q (called Care/Sat) questionnaire developed earlier by Larson. They found three subscales of the tool: benign neglect, enabling, and assistive. In this study, patients in a community hospital perceived less benign neglect, more enabling, and more satisfaction with their care than did patients in teaching hospitals. These authors defined caring as intentional actions that convey physical care and emotional concern and promote a sense of safeness and security in another. They found six themes of caring: accessibility, anticipation, comfort, trusting, relationships, explanation and facilitation, monitoring and follow-through. They concluded, "This instrument, developed and refined in a series of research studies, provides a patient satisfaction measure that is based on the theoretical premise of caring at the behavioral level of nursing practice" (p. 705). In this study, there were two goals: to study the patients and to validate the questionnaire. The description of caring was very complete, and the questionnaire performed well.

The research about caring has some inconsistencies and some similarities. Many studies were done by qualitative methods. These studies did not discuss their methodologies in many cases, so it was hard to evaluate the validity of those studies. Since caring is a relationship and had not been researched much before 1980, it was expected that most studies would be qualitative. The studies, for the most part, involved patient-nurse relationships, and the results were often specific to their population. I found it interesting to read the many words and phrases that defined caring. The descriptions of caring were not always the same, but many had the same basic meanings. A consistent theme was the need to include both knowledge and skills in interpersonal relationships. There were studies that involved quantitative questionnaires developed by the researchers. Wolf (1986) developed the Caring Behaviors Inventory (CBI), which identified ten words or phrases that related to caring behaviors. She did reliability measures to confirm the questionnaire's measurements. Larson (1987) developed the Care Q and Care/Sat and did rigorous validity and reliability measures. Her Care/Sat questionnaire has twenty-nine items that are behaviors related to caring. The other quantitative study about caring was done by me in 1989. I developed the Nyberg Caring Assessment Scale, which did not measure behaviors but rather it identified twenty caring attributes that are more attitude- and belief-based. I would like to present the study here as an example of how a concept such as caring can be studied in a quantitative way. The study will be discussed as it appeared in the *Journal of Nursing Administration* in May 1990. The article has been abridged because the introductory material has already been discussed in this book, but it includes all of the information about the research study.

The Research Study[*]

My study explored caring and nurses' reactions to the economic changes of the recent past. The study included 2,793 nurses from seven hospitals in a western state. A total of 350 questionnaires (50 for each hospital) were sent to randomly selected nurses on staff at various hospitals. There were 135 questionnaires returned (38.57 percent).

Interviews were conducted with the nurse executives of each hospital. The executives were asked to define the characteristics of their hospital and describe their impressions about human care and economics. Their organizations varied from profit to nonprofit, private to public, urban to suburban, teaching to nonteaching, 125 beds to 400 beds. When asked about human care and economics, the nurse executives agreed that it is important for the two concepts to be viewed as interdependent; human care is the goal of nursing, but economics cannot be ignored. The nurse administrators also identified the nursing shortage as a serious problem for the delivery of patient care. One nurse administrator proposed a model that placed caring as the mission of the hospital with economics, research, management, and education as supporting facets.

A questionnaire was developed (Figure 10.1) that identified caring attributes from a variety of previous authors (Mayeroff 1971, Noddings 1984, Watson 1979, Gaut 1983, and Nyberg, unpublished). The attributes included "deep respect for the needs of others," "expresses positive and negative feelings," "believes that others have potential which can be achieved," and "remains committed to a continuing relationship." A series of questions regarding Nyberg's attributes of caring were asked: "How important are the attributes (ideal scale)? How often do you use these attributes in your practice (actual scale)? How often does your supervisor use the caring attributes (supervisor scale)? How have the attributes changed in the past five years (five-year scale)?"

In addition to the Nyberg caring attributes, Larson's (1984) Care Q tool was used. That tool focuses on caring behaviors such as "checks on

---

* Reprinted with permission from *The Journal of Nursing Administration*, Vol. 20, No. 5, pp. 13–18. This is an excerpt from the article entitled "The Effects of Care and Economics on Nursing Practice."

Nyberg Caring Assessment Scale

Are these caring attributes things you actually use in your day-to-day practice?	Cannot use in practice	Occasionally use in practice	Sometimes use in practice	Often use in practice	Always use in practice
Do you:	1	2	3	4	5
1. Have deep respect for the needs of others.					
2. Not give up hope for others.					
3. Remain sensitive to the needs of others.					
4. Communicate a helping, trusting attitude toward others.					
5. Express positive and negative feelings.					
6. Solve problems creatively.					
7. Understand that spiritual forces contribute to human care.					
8. Consider relationships before rules.					
9. Base decisions on what is best for the people involved.					
10. Understand thoroughly what situations mean to people.					
11. Go beyond the superficial to know people well.					
12. Implement skills and techniques that will accomplish goals.					
13. Choose tactics that will accomplish goals.					
14. Give full consideration to situational factors.					
15. Focus on helping others grow.					
16. Take time for personal needs and growth.					
17. Allow time for personal needs and growth.					
18. Remain committed to a continuing relationship.					
19. Listen carefully and be open to feedback.					
20. Believe that others have a potential that can be achieved.					

FIGURE 10.1

A Caring Approach in Nursing Administration

patient frequently," "suggests questions for the patient to ask his/her doctor," "sits down with the patient," and "knows how to give shots, IVs, etc."

A pilot study of the questionnaire was conducted using graduate nursing students at the state university. Reliability for the subscales of the questionnaire (ideal, actual, five-year, supervisor, Care Q) ranged from 0.87 to 0.98 using Cronbach's alpha coefficient. The reliability for the questionnaire for the study population ranged from 0.85 to 0.97, indicating excellent reliability for the whole questionnaire.

Mean scores and standard deviations were calculated to determine how the respondents rated the subscales of the questionnaires. Results indicated that nurses view caring as "very important" (score of 4.1 out of 5), that they use the attributes "often" (score of 3.9), that they practice the attributes "about the same" as five years ago (score of 3), and that supervisors scored lower than the nurses themselves (score of 3.4). The standard deviation for the supervisor scale was highest, indicating extreme scores; some supervisors were rated very high and others were scored very low. The Care Q caring behaviors were also practiced "often" (score of 4.0).

A two-factor analysis of variance was conducted to determine whether there were significant differences between the subscales of the questionnaire and whether these differences were consistent across hospitals. It was found that there were significant differences between ideal, actual, five-year scale, and the supervisor scale.

Finally, the correlation between caring scores and economic indicators was calculated. Two types of economic indicators were used: total nursing hours per patient-day, and total nursing hours per patient-day adjusted by case-mix index. The case-mix index is a Medicare designation reflecting how many acutely ill patients are in each hospital. Adjusting nursing hours by case-mix attempts to control the extraneous variable of patient acuity. The correlation coefficient for the total nursing hours with caring scores was 0.59 ($p=0.07$). The correlation coefficient for adjusted nursing hours and caring scores was 0.73 ($p=0.04$). This indicates that hospitals who used higher numbers of nurses per patient exhibited higher actual caring scores.

At the end of the questionnaire, four open-ended questions were asked. The first two questions concerned economics and the last two questions concerned human care.

The economic questions were answered very negatively and it was apparent that the vast majority of the study participants believed that current economic pressures are making it much harder to provide adequate human care. There were dozens of comments about how sick patients have become and how frustrating it is for nurses not to have time to meet patients' needs. The participants cited short-staffing as a major issue and said that administrators (including nursing administrators) are more interested in money than in what happens to patients. One nurse said that the emphasis on money is "foreign and disgusting" and several nurses expressed feeling desperately rushed, having time to do "only the essentials," and feeling "more distant from patients."

The last two questions addressed human care and elicited very different answers. Nurses understand and value human care as:

- providing care that pays tribute to the dignity of the patient
- being able to laugh and cry with patients
- reaching out human to human
- unconditional positive regard
- dealing with the whole person
- being concerned with the betterment of another

When asked how to maintain care, nurses' answers were again warm and personal:

- developing trusting relationships
- involving the family
- facilitating opportunities for growth
- being an example to other professionals
- being honest and knowing your limits

Most nurses seem to accept caring responsibilities with a great deal of pride and understanding. One nurse said that "nursing practice must have as its foundation the caring aspect of art/science. It is caring that makes nursing unique and essential."

Recommendations

An important overall conclusion from the study is that economics and human care are interrelated forces in today's hospital environment. Nurses' ability to provide care is dependent on economic resources. However, the study also showed that the hospital's ability to provide high levels of human care, this ensuring economic viability, is dependent on nurses.

Further research is recommended to enhance the reliability of the tool and to validate the correlation between human care and economics. Limitations of the study relate to the geographic distribution and the moderate response rate of the questionnaire. A replicate study on a national basis with better follow-up to enhance the findings would be needed to generalize the findings. Organizational assessments should be done to attempt to identify other barriers to human care and more efficient means of providing that care.

Human care is the hope for nursing. Although the current economic environment is severe, this study showed that nurses continue to see caring as important and they still use caring attributes and behaviors in their work. It was interesting to note that, although the economic resources (nursing hours per patient-day) varied by over 200 percent in the study, the ideal and actual measurements of caring did not vary significantly across hospitals. This suggests that human caring is universally seen by nurses as their purpose and their achievement. Nurses' efforts to emphasize human care in their practice should be supported and rewarded.

This study also highlights the Lockian paradox of individual freedom versus the necessity of organization. In 1690 John Locke wrote that the enjoyment of total freedom is uncertain, and therefore people choose to join societies that restrict individual freedom in exchange for security. Morgan (1986) wrote about restrictions imposed by organizations on their employees. Nurses must practice under a certain amount of restrained individual freedom as long as they work in organizations and cultures. This does not mean that human care should be neglected because of economics. It does mean, however, that nurses should recognize that not all of the factors surrounding patient care are under the control of nursing. Nurses must accept the constraints while working optimally within them. As one nurse said, "The greater the economic pressure becomes, the more vigilant we must be to preserve human caring on a high level and the more creative we must be to allow it to continue in the face of greater and greater limitations of time and resources."

The next administrative recommendation is that nursing administrators maintain an awareness of the quality imperative. Donabedian (1984) reminds us that, in the final analysis, there is no substitute for professional commitment and accountability. Quality of care remains our highest mission. One nurse in the study wrote that, in her hospital, she had been told to provide safe care rather than quality care. This is alarming because maintaining a quality approach in any business is necessary (Iacocca, 1988). The problem currently seems to be that nurses are frustrated because they feel obligated to meet more and more patient needs with fewer and fewer resources. Identifying more efficient ways of providing care is a must, but sometimes the economics of an organization outstrip efficiency maneuvers. In such a case, nursing services should be defined by nurses in the organization in such a way that dollar cuts will translate into service cuts. If economic resources make it difficult to allow optimal patient care goals, the nurse administrator has a responsibility to obtain more resources from the organization or else work with nurses to redefine what expectations are realistic within given constraints. In this way, nurses' work is defined in such a manner that they can feel pride in the quality of the care that they do provide.

The last recommendation concerns nursing's place in the organization. Nurses in this study indicated that they felt controlled by "the system" and unable to effect decisions in the organization. Two ways in which nursing's participation in the organization can be enhanced are changing the image of the nursing administrators and changing the organization design.

Porter-O'Grady (1986) wrote that it is time for the relationship between nurses and nurse administrators to change. The nurse administrators of the future need to view themselves as facilitators rather than bosses. For nurses to feel they have input in organizational decisions, they need to view their nurse administrators as colleagues in the effort to provide optimal nursing care.

Changes in the formal organizational structure can also enhance nurses' perceptions of their effectiveness within the health care organization. Such systems as shared governance and participative management give nurses opportunities to become a part of the decision-making process. It is no longer appropriate for one nurse—the chief executive—to be the only nurse's voice in the organization. Rather, a philosophy of participation can be implemented that allows many nurses to speak for patient care and nursing's interests.

Conclusion

Economics and human care must be viewed as interrelated forces within today's hospital environment. Economics was seen by nurses in this study as a constraining force in health care while human care was recognized as nursing's responsibility and goal. Ray's (1989) theory of bureaucratic caring suggests that caring exists in the hospital in a variety of forms. Tending to economics is a form of caring, in that it secures the organization's ability to support human care as it is expressed by nurses to patients. While it is clear that economic adjustments are necessary to maintain the viability of hospital organizations, the product of human care must be protected and encouraged for the welfare of patients, nurses, and the hospital. Wisdom for the nurse administrator is in recognizing the realities of both human care and economics and integrating them into a system where the goals of patient care and organizational survival are mutually supportive.

Discussion of the Research Study

The reason to read about my quantitative study of caring is to get a feel for such a study. It also offers some insights about caring that the study illuminated. It is important to know where the attributes came from. In the case of the Larson Care/Sat and Wolfe's CBI tools, it says that the authors developed them using other nurses as experts, and literature. In my tool, the items were quite literally taken from the literature. The first seven items came from Watson's carative factors, the next three were from Noddings' work, others were from Gaut and Mayeroff, and the last five were from my own work as published in the article "The Element of Caring in Nursing Administration" (see chapter three). Still, I was concerned about whether the items were important ones to nurses at all levels of the organization. That is why the first thing I asked on the questionnaire was, "How important are these attributes to you?" The answer was a strong one: the nurses said that the items were "very important." The Nyberg Caring Assessment Scale has been used in many other studies. The scores remain strong and the reliabilities high. The most important difference in the three quantitative scales is that the Nyberg scale measures attributes, not behaviors. The Larson scale measures mostly behaviors and the CBI is a mixture of attitudes, beliefs, and behaviors. It is important for researchers to study each tool and give some thought to what they are trying to measure before choosing a questionnaire.

It is important to note that my study included a qualitative piece (the open-ended questions), and that I received a great deal of information from them. The conclusions at the end of the study were drawn from both the qualitative and quantitative data. This study was done in 1989. I am afraid that the frustration about economics is even worse today. I believe also that caring is still desired, practiced, and appreciated.

Qualitative Research on Caring

Now, I want to outline a qualitative study that is in progress as an example of what the differences are. At a local hospital, a small committee was given the task of implementing caring (focused on Watson's theory) on a pediatric oncology unit. The first question was, "Do the nurses on this unit *want* to implement a caring philosophy and modalities?" Once it was ascertained that they did, the researchers (of whom I am one) began to think of how to structure such a task. The nursing executive at the hospital is very supportive of nursing research, so it was decided that the program would be a research project as well as a nursing care delivery project.

We began by having several hours of discussion about the unit and the task ahead. The research team all agreed that we wanted to use qualitative research methods, because our goal was to improve care for the patients, and we felt that we would get more and richer data from a qualitative study. At the same time, the administrator wanted to track costs and examine some other variables regarding contextual variables. Context was defined as a general setting or set of circumstances in which a particular event or situation occurs. Examples of contextual variables are market forces, economic constraints, organizational structure, core values, technology, and management direction. In most clinical studies, no one keeps track of the "side issues," i.e., contextual variables that can affect the study. For example, in one hospital I consulted with, the hospital was sold in the middle of our study. It was difficult to tell what affected what. It was something no one could predict, but we decided it was important to acknowledge the extraneous variable in the results on the study.

So, in effect, our research would be a triangulated qualitative/ quantitative study. First it was decided that we had to define our assumptions and goals for the study. Then we wrote the theoretical base for the study (most of which has been covered in the first three chapters of this book). We then began to discuss the methodology for the study. We read a book by Reason (1988) on human inquiry. We read that it is very important to explore the relationships among the researchers in a research project and even the relationships to those being researched. We examined this closely, and spent specific time getting to know each other.

Reason (1988) believes in process-oriented, action research, which recognizes that the research is performed in the lives of those researched and those doing the research. He believes that such process-oriented research is evolving from a changing paradigm which recognizes that reality cannot be objectively defined. This is in agreement with what I have tried to stress in this book. The new paradigm is based on wholeness and relationships. The research of such a philosophy will be more personally oriented, and the researchers will see themselves as part of the research process.

Reason wrote about "cooperative inquiry," where all those involved in the research are involved in the critical thinking that goes into the study. Another name for cooperative research is participatory research. The emphasis is in establishing a dialogue between researchers and the researched in an attempt to establish relationships of authentic collaboration. The researchers and the researched care for each other, and hierarchy is diminished as much as possible. Another term used for this type of research is action-research. This implies that what is discovered in the research process is put into action instead of in a report that sits in someone's drawer. The action research should be seen as a method of problem solving and planning for new or improved systems.

We decided that the immediate method of study would be focus groups. These are carefully set up groups that have insight into the problem being studied. For us, that meant we would construct groups of nurses on the study unit, patients on the unit, families of children that were cared for on the study unit, non-nurse providers from the unit, and a final group that would be the research group itself. Unfortunately, our funding was restricted to looking only at the effect our caring education had on nurses, so the focus groups were done only with nurses.

Focus groups were first used by marketing specialists in industry to assess consumer's opinions about new products. More recently, focus groups have been used in service organizations such as hospitals. The groups are conducted by a facilitator, but the emphasis is on a loose, free-flowing conversation where participants can feel safe to really discuss the topic under study. Focus groups often provide a great deal of information and lend themselves to studies of problems that need in-depth investigation. The moderator creates a permissive atmosphere that encourages different perceptions and points of view. After the group meets, the researcher analyzes the discussion to try to identify trends and patterns in the communications of participants. The focus group method allows much more personal information than other quantitative methods. Kingry et al. (1990) suggest that focus groups can be used along with other quantitative measures to increase the richness of the total research data.

We felt very excited about using focus groups, seeing them as the best source of information about how nurses feel about the treatment they give to children with life-threatening illnesses. Since our topic of interest was caring, we planned to use a few open-ended questions to get the participants to talk about caring as they saw it in this population. The moderators for the groups were to be the researchers, and there would always be two researchers at each group so that they could validate with each other about the information they heard.

The implementation phase of the project consisted of three objectives:

1. To present the philosophy of caring in such a way that the nurses' perceptions of themselves as persons and care-givers will become aligned with the philosophy.

2. To teach specific caring/healing modalities (such as relaxation and imaging, music therapy, massage, therapeutic touch, etc.) that nurses will use in their everyday work with patients.

3. To create structures, such as new documentation, to encourage and validate integration of these practices.

To meet these aims, there will be an educational intervention which will:
1. didactically teach nurses the philosophy and theories of caring/healing and

relationship-centered care; 2. use role modeling, storytelling, and patient interview to translate the theory to lived experience that nurses can use in their care-giving; 3. actually teaching the nurses how to do extended nursing healing/caring practices including massage, relaxation, guided imagery, therapeutic touch, and music therapy; 4. provide on-unit assistance for a three-month implementation phase where nurses will use the caring modalities with support available to them on-call from the project director.

For the evaluation process there will be a repeat of the preimplementation measures, including focus groups, the Nyberg Caring Assessment Scale, the Contextual Variable questionnaire, cost analysis, and chart reviews. The evaluation will take place six months after the teaching sessions.

The anticipated outcomes involve an improved relationship between nurses and patients, and less suffering for the patients. To measure such a nebulous outcome, qualitative measures will be of utmost importance. The researchers will keep logs of the changes they see happening, and the nurses' focus groups will give a great deal of information regarding the effects of the project.

Although this study is in the beginning phase of implementation, it is easy to see how it will differ from a quantitative study. Since caring is so subjective, the study seems subjective, but it is likely to uncover a great deal of very important information about implementing caring as philosophy and modalities. Everyone in the study will be asked to share their feelings about the study, and those feelings will be important for nurses in other studies as caring is implemented.

The Importance of Research in Caring

These two studies are examples of research in relationship to caring. It has been said that nursing is an art and a science. Caring is the art portion of nursing. It is important to study this phenomenon to ensure that it remains an important and validated part of nursing. When one is nursing, the last thing he/she wants to do is take the time to study it. It is like that with caring. We want to do it, not study it! But research is an important part of nursing's future, so study it we must.

References

Blegen, M. A. and C. Boode (1994). Interactive process of conducting and utilizing research in nursing service administration. *The Journal of Nursing Administration* 24 (9): 24–28.

Bostrom, J. and L. Wise (1994). Closing the gap between research and practice. *Journal of Nursing in Administration* 24 (5): 22–27.

Bower, F. (1994). Outcomes must be the focus. *Reflections* (Fall): 4.

Breitmayer, B. J. and K. A. Knafl (1994). Triangulation in quantitative and qualitative research. *Image: Journal of Nursing Scholarship* 25 (3): 237–244.

Brett, J. L. (1989). Indicators of quality care. In B. Henry, C. Arndt, A. Marriner-Tomey, and M. Divincenti, eds., *Dimensions of Nursing Administration*. Boston: Blackwell Scientific Publications, pp. 353–371.

Brooten, D. and M. Naylor (1995). Nurses' effect on changing patient outcomes. *Image* 27 (2): 95–97.

Brown, L. (1986). The experience of care: Patient perspectives. *Topics in Clinical Nursing* 8 (2): 56–62.

Cronin, S. N. (1993). Identifying nursing research priorities in an acute care hospital. *Journal of Nursing Administration* 23 (11): 58–62.

Donabedian, A. (1984). Quality, cost, and cost containment. *Nursing Outlook* 32 (3): 142–145.

Dzurec, L. C. (1993). The nature of inquiry: Linking quantitative and qualitative research. *Advances in Nursing Sciences* 16 (1): 73–77.

Gaut, D. (1983). A theoretic description of caring as action. In M. Leininger, ed., *Care: The Essence of Nursing and Health*. Detroit: Wayne State University Press.

Hegyvary, S. T. (1991). Outcome research: Integrating nursing practice into the world view, USHHS; NIH. Patient Outcomes research: Examining the effectiveness of nursing practice. Proceedings of a Conference Sponsored by the National Center for Nursing Research.

Hinshaw, A. S. (1989) Programs of nursing research for nursing administration. In Henry, Arndt, Devincenti, Marriner-Tomey, eds., *Dimensions of Nursing Administration*. Boston: Blackwell Publishing Company, pp. 251–265.

Hinshaw, A. S. and C. H. Smeltzer (1987). Research challenges and programs for practice settings. *The Journal of Nursing Administration* 17 (7, 8): 20–26.

Hutchison, C. P. and R. T. Bahr, Sr. (1991). Types and meanings of caring behaviors among elderly nursing home residents. *Image: The Journal of Nursing Scholarship* 23 (2): 85–88.

Iaccoca, L. (1988). *Talking Straight*. New York: Bantum Books.

Kingry, M. J., L. B. Tiedje, and L. L. Friedman (1990). Focus groups: A research technique for nursing. *Nursing Research* 39 (2): 124–125.

Larson, P. J. (1987). Comparison of cancer patients and professional nurses' perceptions of important nursing caring behaviors. *Heart and Lung* 16 (2): 187–193.

———. (1984). Important nurse caring behaviors perceived by patients with cancer. *Oncology Nursing Forum* 11 (6): 46–50.

Larson P. J. and S. F. Ferhetich (1993). Patient's satisfaction with nurses' caring during hospitalization. *Western Journal of Nursing Research* 15 (6): 690–707.

Mayer, D. K. (1986). Cancer patients and families perceptions of nurse caring behaviors. *Topics in Clinical Nursing* 8 (2): 63–69.

Mayeroff, M. (1971). *On Caring*. New York: Barnes and Noble Books.

Miller, K. (1994). Assessing the context of care in patient outcomes research. In J. Fitzpatrick, J. Stevenson, and N. Polis, eds., *Nursing Research and Its Utilization*. New York: Springer Co. pp. 107–116.

Morgan, G. (1986). *Images of Organizations*. Beverly Hills, CA: Sage Publishers.

Noddings, N. (1984). *Caring*. Berkeley, CA: University of California Press.

Nyberg, J. (1990). The effects of caring and economies on nursing practice. *The Journal of Nursing Administration* 20 (5): 13–18.

Polit, D. F., and B. P. Hungler, (1983). *Nursing Research: Principles and Methods*. Philadelphia: J. B. Lippincott.

Porter-O'Grady, T. (1986). *Creative Nursing Administration: Participative Management for the 21st Century*. Rockville, MD: Aspen Publications.

Ray, M. A. (1987). Technological caring: A new model in critical care. *Dimensions of Critical Care* 6 (3): 166–173.

———. (1989). The theory of bureaucratic caring for nursing practice in the organizational culture. *Nursing Administration Quarterly* 13 (2): 31–42.

Reason, P. (1988). *Human Inquiry in Action*. London: Sage Publication.

Rieman, D. J. (1986). Noncaring and caring in the clinical setting: Patient descriptions. *Topics in Clinical Nursing* 8 (2): 30–36.

Rizzo, J. A., M. P. Gilman, C. A. Mersmann, (1994). Facilitating care delivery redesign using measures of unit culture and work characteristics. *The Journal of Nursing Administration* 24 (5): 32–37.

Schultz, P. R. and K. L. Miller (1994). Nursing administration research, part one: Pluralities of persons. *Research on Nursing Care Delivery.* pp. 133–158.

Shiber, S. and E. Larson (1991). Evaluation of the quality of caring: Structure, process, and outcome. *Holistic Nursing Practice* 5 (3): 57–66.

Smith, M. (1993). The contribution of nursing theory to nursing administration. *Image: Journal of Nursing Scholarship* 25 (1): 63–67.

Sperhac, A. M., S. A. Hass, and J. O. O'Malley (1994). Supporting nursing research: A representative program. *The Journal of Nursing Administration* 24 (5): 28–31.

Swanson, K. M. (1990). Providing care in the NICU: Sometimes an act of love. *Advances in Nursing Science* 13 (1): 60–73.

Swanson-Kaufman, K. M. (1986). Caring in the instance of unexpected pregnancy loss. *Topics in Clinical Nursing* 8 (2): 37–46.

Valentine, K. (1989). Caring is more than kindness: Modeling its complexities. *The Journal of Nursing Administration* 19 (11): 28–34.

Waltz, C. F. and O.L. Strickland (1988). Measurement of nursing outcomes: Volume I. *Measuring Client Outcomes*. New York: Springer.

Watson, J. (1985). *Human Science and Human Care*. Norwalk, CT: Appleton-Century-Crofts.

————. (1979). *Nursing: The Philosophy and Science of Caring*. Boulder, CO: Colorado Associated University Press.

Wolf, Z. R. (1986). The caring concept and nurse identified caring behaviors. *Topics in Clinical Nursing* 8(2): 84–93.

Wolf, Z. R., E. R Giardino, F. A. Osborne, and M. S. Ambrose (1994). Dimensions of nursing caring. *Image: The Journal Of Nursing Scholarship* 23 (2): 107–111.

Chapter Ten

Organizational Effectiveness and Quality Management

Organizations exist for a purpose. All organizations have goals that they try to meet. That means they must have a way to judge whether they are meeting their goals or not. That judgment can be termed organizational effectiveness or quality management. Some organizations have well-defined goals—making judgment of effectiveness easy—and some organizations seem to just run every day with no sense of purpose.

Organizational Effectiveness

Organizational effectiveness can mean various things to different people, in the organization and outside of it. For example, employees may have the goal of organizational survival so they can keep working, while those coming into the organization as patients will feel that the organization is effective if they get well. Some measures of organizational effectiveness include:

1. Goal attainment (assuming someone has defined the goals).

2. Meeting standards (the problem is in defining the standards).

3. Output vs. input (does the organization produce output that exceeds input resulting in a profit?).

4. Survival of the organization (some say that the only measure of success is whether the organization survives).

5. Satisfied employees (some patients and managers couldn't care less if the employees are happy).

6. Meet society's needs (something few organizations think about).

In a health care organization, there are many interested people who may all have different goals. The doctors want a workshop that makes it easiest to care for their patients. The administrators want an organization that "runs well" and makes a profit. The board of directors want to make a profit, but may also be quite aware of the societal obligation. The community wants a place that is convenient and gives "good care." The employees want good pay, a nice work environment, and the resources that allow them to do their best work. The suppliers want an organization that orders lots of expensive equipment and pays its bills on time. The payers (usually insurance companies) want good care, but they want it to be cheap—they would prefer to not have their clients in health care organizations at all. The government (who now pays about 40 percent of health care bills) wants an accredited organization that will accept their payment. Indeed, organizational effectiveness is at best an elusive concept, since all of these wants are legitimate. Also, in health care, there is no margin for error—we must do everything right the first time or our customers may have no ability to come back!

Scott (1981) wrote about organizational effectiveness, and he defines three types of organizations. The rational organization is like the bureaucracy we have discussed. He says that a rational system's measures of effectiveness are attainment of goals, output, and efficiency. The natural system conforms to our description of the human relations structure. In these organizations, effectiveness is survival, so that employees maintain a place to work, and employee satisfaction. The open-system organization is like the newer forms we have defined. The goals of these systems include being successful in a highly interdependent environment. In effect, the goal of the organization is the ability to exploit its environment so that it can be a top-notch organization that meets the goals of all the people and systems that depend on it. I do not think we consider enough the organizational effectiveness of creating a value to the community. In my view, health care's goal is to meet the needs of the community for health care. Effectiveness would be a healthy community.

Jackson, Morgan, and Paolilla (1986) wrote about the importance of measuring organizational effectiveness. They believe that we must differentiate between effectiveness and efficiency. Efficiency means using the lowest cost of producing a good or service. While efficiency is one measure of effectiveness, it is only one, and other goals must not be subordinated to efficiency. The most obvious other goal is effectiveness, which is the best possible result. Jackson, Morgan, and Paolilla note that there are short-term and long-term indicators of effectiveness: the short-term indicators are production, efficiency, and satisfaction. The intermediate indicators are adaptiveness and development. The ultimate indicator is survival. Again, I think survival is not a good measure of effectiveness. There are some procedures that have better results if done many times (heart surgery, for example). The organization that does only a few each year cannot be as efficient or effective. This is where it depends on your position as to your measure of effectiveness. For the community as a whole, effectiveness may mean that the organization does not survive. Jackson, Morgan, and Paolilla wrote about why it is important to study effectiveness:

1. To demonstrate to others that the organization is worthwhile.

2. To determine if it is moving in the right direction.

3. To determine whether the organization is satisfying the needs of the public.

4. To justify expenditures.

5. To determine costs.

6. To obtain evidence of program effectiveness.

7. To gain support for expansion.

8. To compare programs.

These authors also define when not to evaluate effectiveness:

1. If costs of the evaluation are too high.

2. When the current program is the only way.

3. When the program is obviously desired in spite of its effectiveness.

4. When change would be too disruptive.

These organizational theorists leave me with the feeling that they view the organization as an inanimate object that you can just look at from afar and decide how things are going. We know from working in them that this is not the case. Everything is complex and interdependent, and measuring anything depends on the people doing the evaluation and what they are evaluating. Health care is not very measurable at times, and it is hard to take the time of the professionals to do the evaluation. I can understand effectiveness better from the writings of Bracy et al. (1991), who wrote about "managing from the heart." They say that the first step is for managers to plan for, train, and motivate employees within the perspective of their company's mission or vision. They believe that a company cannot maintain high-quality people, products, and profits unless it is managed with compassion and caring. Managing from the heart is the way caring and respect can be spread throughout the business world. That is done by listening to what your people say:

1. Please don't make me wrong, even if you disagree.
2. Hear me and understand me.
3. Tell me the truth with compassion.
4. Remember to look for my loving intentions.
5. Acknowledge the greatness within me.

(p. 13)

To me, treating employees in this caring manner does more for quality than all the measurements you can think of.

Quality Management

Whether we like it or not, measuring organizational effectiveness is an important undertaking. We would like to think that we don't need to measure—that we do everything well all the time—but such is not the case. In nursing (and most businesses now) the emphasis is on *quality management*. There are all sorts of acronyms for quality: QA = quality assurance or assessment; QI = quality improvement; TQI = total quality improvement; QM = quality management; TQM = total quality management. Each may have a slightly different emphasis, but they all mean that someone is watching out for quality.

In the organization where I worked, quality assurance was just starting to gain attention when I became an administrator. Until then, the

A Caring Approach in Nursing Administration

Joint Commission for Accreditation of Hospitals (JCAH) had required that doctors and nurses do quarterly chart audits to improve the quality of care. That was done, but it was mostly done as an extra chore, and the impact was limited.

Soon after I was hired as the associate director of nursing, I was sent to a workshop about developing a quality assurance program. Then, I was assigned to start such a program in our hospital. One thing that impressed me at the conference were the quality assurance nurses, who said that they were very frustrated because everyone at their hospitals was saying things like, "You're the quality assurance nurse, so you are responsible for quality." That seemed unfair to me. I understood the need to have specific quality assurance projects, but I felt it was wrong for any one person to be responsible for quality.

As a new administrator, I was trying very hard to work with staff nurses on projects. It seemed to me that the only way to have a good quality assurance program was to make it something for all nurses. We formed a quality assurance committee that had one staff nurse from each nursing unit. I chaired the meetings at first, and we tried to find things to investigate that had relevance to us. We knew we had to meet the JCAH requirements, but we did things the way we thought were best, and assumed that, if we really tried to improve, our efforts would have meaning to us and the JCAH.

In time, the committee was turned over to the staff nurses to run, with administration being consultants to them. After we had a plan for the nursing department as a whole, we progressed to unit-based quality assurance, and we had poster sessions once a year to display our projects. We never achieved perfection, but we made progress on problems that had plagued us for years (such as medication errors and patient falls). We did have a quality assurance nurse, but we titled her position as the "quality assessment coordinator," and she too was to help the staff, not be responsible for quality. The other group we needed to get involved was the unit nurse managers. We discussed with them regularly how their units were doing with quality assurance, and told them that their units' activities in quality assurance would affect their personal performance appraisals. This was important because the staff nurses had a very hard time getting anything accomplished unless the nurse manager was very supportive.

Let's go back and consider the quality coordinators of today. Megel and Elrod (1993) wrote about the experience of QA/QI nurse professionals. They say that with the current emphasis on quality in health care organizations, there are new roles for professionals. With new computerized methods and changing regulations, the responsibility of QA/QI nurses is increasing. Now these nurses are responsible not just for nursing quality, they are getting new responsibilities throughout the organization. Some times this sets up conflict in the organization. Conflict, however, is considered normal, not negative, and can lead to creative tension, which can serve as a catalyst for change. These authors did a study of ethical and interpersonal conflicts of QI nurses. It was a descriptive study involving nine participants. They found that the QI nurses experienced both types of conflicts. Interpersonal conflicts were defined as disagreement among two or more individuals involving incompatible concerns. Ethical conflicts occurred when it was not clear whether a particular action was ethically justifiable and there were overriding concerns in determining the "right" thing to do. Most of the nurses used the justice perspective, where traditional ethical principles such as confidentiality, fairness, truth telling, autonomy, and patients' rights to quality of care prevail. A caring perspective was also identified, which emphasized understanding and connectedness, avoiding hurting others, and retaining relationships. The nurses identified interpersonal conflicts involving power and authority (for example, "I feel that as nurse QA/QI coordinator I have limited ability to push an issue"). Ethical issues included deciding when data regarding quality of care and staff performance should be shared with others for learning purposes or for improvement of patient care. The authors concluded, "We believe strategies from both the caring and justice perspectives could be helpful in resolving ethical and values conflicts that arise between QA/QI professionals and staff and administrators" (p. 16). From the justice perspective, it is important to be objective, fair, and confidential in regard to all policies and standards of practice. From the caring perspective, it is important to listen to and understand the other's point of view and work with others in ways that facilitate the development and maintenance of interpersonal relationships.

Well, the years have passed, and we now have all sorts of quality management techniques. Quality has almost become a buzzword, but many organizations are working hard to improve quality in their organizations.

A Caring Approach in Nursing Administration

Quality is no longer just the problem of doctors and nurses, it is the expectation of every department. I know nurses still sometimes feel that it is just one more paper job that detracts them from patient care, but it is important, and we can be proud that nursing took up the quality banner long before other departments. This book is about caring, and nothing is more caring than trying to make our nursing systems as high quality as possible.

Price (1993) wrote that quality is a major issue facing the delivery of health services today. The need for nurses to understand and deliver quality care is congruent with patients' expectations and with the nursing ideology of client-centered care. Indeed, quality of nursing care is frequently a major determinant of client satisfaction of their whole hospital stay. This author did a grounded theory study with four participants (parents of hospitalized children) asking the question, "What does quality nursing care mean to parents of hospitalized children?" The study found that parents' experiences with quality nursing care involved a process of maneuvering (where the parent tries to help with the care so the nurses will have more time for their child), a process of knowing (they perceived that it required time on the nurses' part), and finally a positive relationship (where the parents' presence was acknowledged, the nurses' skills were trustworthy, and the parents felt comfortable and listened to). Quality care meant having the needs of the child and parent met. There was a basic expectation that the nurses could use the machines and equipment. Quality care was perceived as the nurse being focused on meeting non-technical needs such information-giving, and a positive reciprocal interaction between nurses and the child and parent. Quality nursing care involves a process of patient, family, and nurse interaction that ultimately results in the satisfaction of biopsychosocial needs of the parent and child. This seems to me to be a very balanced view of quality. It speaks of the conflict from the last chapter about technical skills and interpersonal skills. Price's study affirms Watson's view of skills and knowledge being foundational expectations of caring.

Greeneich (1993) wrote about the link between new and returning business and quality care. She found that quality nursing care was the key to overall patient satisfaction. She suggests that, in the twentieth century, the patient needs to be seen as the decision maker, with the nurse as a facilitator. Partnership is espoused as the appropriate nurse-patient relationship. The match between patient expectations and nursing actually received is expressed as patient satisfaction, and patient satisfaction has been widely adopted as an indicator of quality of care. Greeneich found that caring was a unique professional characteristic connected to patient satisfaction. She found that, in many cases, patients had a critical juncture—a nursing care event that occurs when the patient is most vulnerable—that left a strong lasting impression, good or bad. The nurse administrator can have a big impact on developing a patient-driven system by being committed to staff, procurement of information and education, and development of a quality, service-oriented culture.

Ludwig-Beymer et al. (1993) also wrote that nursing satisfaction is a measure of total patient satisfaction. In contrast, failing to meet the customer's expectation of quality will result in customer dissatisfaction and is usually an indicator of poor quality. These authors believe that health care consumers are very able to define the care they receive. I have some trouble with such sweeping statements, because I think there are times when the patients do not know when a procedure or treatment is of high quality. I believe that we should pay strong attention to patients' perceptions, but our job includes treating some things the patient does not understand.

Ludwig-Beymer et.al. did a grounded theory study about quality care by analysis of unsolicited letters, patient satisfaction questionnaires filled out at time of discharge, and questionnaires mailed after discharge. They discovered two categories of patient perception: global experience and quality nursing care. Five global experiences were identified: 1.attachment (the patient wants to keep up with the organization after discharged); 2. community (experience the institution's service obligation); 3. consistency (there was coordination and teamwork across department and time); 4. caring (comfort, caring, activity); and 5. life events (specific critical events). Quality nursing care experience was characterized by patients as a "calling of the head (capable, efficient, knowledgeable, hard working)" and a "calling of the heart (caring, respect, enthusiastic, going the extra mile" (p. 48). I think this is a beautiful way to describe nursing caring. Nurses need to pay attention to these characterizations. While we many times measure quality by mortality, morbidity, and readmissions, we should pay attention to the patients' perceptions of caring of the head and caring of the heart.

Thurston, Watson, and Reimer (1993) wrote about the difference between quality improvement and research. They believe that they are not the same, although they may be closely linked. Research is necessary to discover new methods of providing care or to confirm existing practice. Quality improvement attempts to demonstrate that expected standards and quality of care or service are provided. Quality improvement projects are generally approved by department heads, while research needs broader approval to address scientific rigor and ethical considerations. In my opinion, research and quality improvement are more similar than different. Research usually has more rigorous measurements, but many good quality improvement projects could easily become research if someone in the organization recognizes that potential, and if resources and time are adequate to allow the research to be set up. I would encourage nurses involved in quality assurance to make as many projects as possible research projects. This adds validity to the projects they do.

Sherman and Malkmus (1994) wrote about integrating QA, TQM, and QI. This was a unit-based project that had the purpose of identifying opportunities for improvement based on customers. However, the unit addressed unit-specific changes to increase staff satisfaction instead of the needs of customers. They conclude that QI is a management style rather than a program or procedure. Success comes from high-level management and staff commitment, enthusiasm generated by TQM/QI and the existence of a well-developed program for QA on the unit. In my experience, nurses at the beginning of our QA program also tended to do projects based more on their needs than the patients', but once someone addressed their needs—even just a little—they then moved on quickly to address patient-centered projects.

Carefoote (1994) wrote about total quality management (TQM) as it is implemented in home care agencies. She says that the term TQM was coined in 1985 by the Naval Air Systems Command. TQM is a management approach to long-term success through customer satisfaction. Its benefits are lower costs, increased revenues, enhanced operations, improvement in clinical outcomes, a way to prove service value, and creation of organizational synergy. This approach sounds like the answer to all organizational problems. I appreciate the emphasis on customer satisfaction, but I wonder if a TQM program can result in all the benefits listed. The navy views TQM as a management process rather than a distinct program. I think it is great for an organization to make quality a central focus, but I think having QA employees can facilitate and coordinate quality assurance projects. The management principles involved in TQM are:

1. The structure and function of the organization consistently supports a consumer-oriented philosophy.

2. The organization must consistently provide services and products of the highest quality.

3. The organization must have adequate human, financial, and physical resources organized to accommodate its stated purpose.

4. The organization must be positioned for long-term viability.

It is important to look for projects that are directly relevant to your agency, that will advance your place in the marketplace, that are highly visible and motivating, and are resolvable within a reasonable time frame. Carefoote says that TQM is meant to become a way of doing things, not another thing to do (I agree with that premise). She suggests that the following questions be asked before TQM is implemented:

1. Who is the customer here?

2. What does he/she need or want from me?

3. How can I exceed their expectations?

4. What is the underlying process or system in question?

5. What data do I need to make a sound decision?

6. How can I empower this individual or group of individuals?

7. How can I build improvement into the process?

Fitzpatrick (1994) says that the Joint Commission of Accreditation of Healthcare Organizations (JCAHO) continues to challenge the executives of health care organizations to focus their energies on accessing, measuring, and improving the structures, processes, and outcomes identified in the JCAHO requirements. We should ask, not just are we doing the right thing, but are we doing the right thing right. We must examine our services in relation to availability, efficacy, appropriateness, timeliness, effectiveness, continuity, safety, efficiency, and respect and caring. When dealing with quality measurement, opportunities for improvement must be viewed in a positive manner. Fitzpatrick notes that every process can be improved; poor outcomes are caused by poor procedures, not poor performance by people. (This may not be true all the time. Some employees can

A Caring Approach in Nursing Administration

perform poorly.) Organizations are challenged to provide high-quality care and work toward improving outcomes and controlling costs. This author feels like innovation in process design becomes the key. In my opinion, this description also encompasses nearly all the obligations for the whole organization. If, indeed, quality becomes everybody's goal, then this is good. But if it is just an expensive, time-consuming project for managers, it could become just another tedious activity. Likewise, if QA is expected to be done by a few people in isolation, it may not be utilized. It seems that QA is in need of specific people and management involvement.

Brett (1989) advocates for outcome measures for quality improvement. She recognizes that outcome measures, in nursing and other departments, are hard to quantify and cannot often be attributed to any one part of care. Therefore, outcome measures by themselves are not sufficient in measuring quality. She suggests outcomes such as patient satisfaction, patient knowledge, functional health status, clinical health status, emotional health status, perceptions of patient/family and doctors and nurses, disposition of patient, negative results or complications, discharge readiness, patient compliance, and appearance of the patient.

Shiber and Larson (1991) wrote about evaluating the quality of nursing care by structure, process, and outcome. An example of structural quality control is the educational experience of the nurse, the organizational structure, and nursing standards of care. Process elements of quality measurement include interpersonal relationships between nurses and patients, nursing knowledge and competencies, and change-of-shift reports. Quality outcome indicators look at what effect the nursing care has on the patient. Examples include growth and development of the patient, ability to cope with illness, ability to get personal needs met, and a perception by patients that they have been well cared for.

Goode (1995) agrees that it is important to look at process and outcomes of care. She recommends measuring the patient outcomes before changing nursing practice, and then remeasuring them after the change is in place. Goode recommends that the results of the measurement should be incorporated into ongoing quality assessment reports so that effects can be examined over time.

The quality assurance program where I worked was based on the structure-process-outcome model. It helped to have that model so that we covered all areas of nurses' work. The QA program gave us direct knowledge about important facets of our work, and it contributed to our knowledge and confidence in the quality of nursing care at our hospital.

Before we leave the subject of quality, we should consider the thoughts of Deming again. He goes beyond pleasing customers to ask, "What does the customer need?" This implies that you plan for things in the future, not just be satisfied with the status quo. Deming (in Lawton, 1993) says that customers only expect what you and your competitors have led them to expect. We must think beyond the now to what will be. Deming says that managers can determine their own future; they can spend their time and energy playing "catch up" or they can proactively seek new ways to create new value for their customers. Organizations must develop ideas that might be of value, work them up to see if they are feasible, and conduct continuous customer research. Deming's philosophy is that, where competition sharpens the saw and tunes us as individuals, cooperation is what will enable us to create strength from diversity and to develop a society and nation that is stronger than any one nationality or culture has been before.

I just do not know what to think of this cooperation vs. competition philosophy. It does seem to be counterproductive to have little cooperation and so much duplication (like in the health care system), but Americans are so competitive! Let's see what else Deming stands for.

Deming's picture of an organization is a network of interconnected processes by which value is created for the customer and continually improved. His goal is to increase the quality of life and economic situation of all. Everyone will eventually lose unless all can win. This is certainly not the way our health care organizations are operating now. The emphasis is on merging into huge conglomerates and competing to the death (literally, because some hospitals will die). Deming says that we should not rely on short-term goals such as monthly or yearly profits, but we should see an organization as a process unfolding through time. The job of management is to create an aim that everyone can believe in and nurture, and that restore the individual's dignity and self-esteem. As far as quality is concerned, Deming would say it is paramount. But, not just QA or QI, but quality as the cornerstone of everyone's work. Quality cannot be split off and managed by a QA coordinator, because quality is everyone's main job. It is not enough to examine quality after the fact; it *is* right to make our systems so good that there are no margins for error.

Strive for every product to be perfect. I like that part of Deming's philosophy, because in patient care there is no margin for error. Deming would say we should constantly improve the work processes to make them perfect, a tall order for sure. One last belief of Deming's concerns how employees are treated. He says that there are no bad people, just bad work processes. When there is meaning to work and the possibility for success, people have all the internal motivation that is needed to do a good job. That is certainly a refreshing change from how people are treated in many competitive businesses. And quality, for Deming, is the natural course of a good organization and good managers.

I really believe, with Deming, that quality cannot be a separate process in an organization. We cannot carve quality out of everybody's job description and give it to a person or a department. It is all right to have special people who work as quality coordinators, but only when everyone understands that quality is everyone's job. Each nurse must be dedicated to quality in their patient care. Every manager must be dedicated to quality with every policy they write and every interaction they have with every employee. Quality is, I think, the job itself.

Quality is clearly a hot topic right now. Some organizations may do very little that looks like the QA/QI programs and yet provide very high quality care. In other organizations, quality management has taken on a life of its own and yet quality is elusive. I would say that all organizations need to consider quality as an important issue, but I do not believe it should be a dominant program where quality becomes the domain of only the QI professionals. Quality is everyone's responsibility and should not be isolated with powerful or powerless QI professionals. I believe that these professionals have much to give when their job is structured well.

In most of the articles we have reviewed, quality and caring are very closely connected. Indeed, two studies have said caring equals patient satisfaction equals quality. To some QI professionals, however, the way they do their job is not always very caring. They may be blaming and heavy-handed to the staff and management nurses. Some seem to get mad at nursing because of the low quality they find, and I agree with that perception at times. Then I think about Benner's *From Novice to Expert,* and I remember that not all nurses are experts, and there will be errors now and then. Even the QI professionals are not always experts in what they do. What this all points to is the importance of caring for everyone involved.

I believe that QI nurses have an excellent forum in which to practice caring. The way that they go about their job can be as role models for caring. In nursing and health care as a whole, we need to treat all our colleagues in the same way that we treat our patients. That's the thing about caring—there is always enough to go around. In fact, the more we give away, the more caring exists in the world.

Quality of care cannot be overrated as an organizational variable. The question is, "Who is responsible for it, and what does the QA/QI nurse do in regard to it?" Until the last few years, this was an internal organizational issue. Now, there are not only nurses in charge of in-house quality, there are many nurses becoming involved with insurance companies and with case management in many different settings. I remain convinced that professionals can never give away their responsibility for providing quality care. But I am also aware that the case manager can spot problems that organizations cannot or do not address. The role of a QI or case manager offers exciting opportunities for many nurses. I am encouraged that so much attention is being given to quality management, because it means that we are not just focused on costs and profits. It reminds us that quality, after all, is our purpose in being care-givers at all.

References

Benner, P. (1984). *From Novice to Expert*. Menlo Park, CA: Addison Wesley.

Bracey, H., J. Rosenblum, A. Sanford, and R. Trueblood (1991). *Managing From the Heart*. New York: Delacorte Press.

Brett, J. L. (1989). Outcome indicators of quality care. *Dimensions of Nursing Administration: Theory, Research, Education, Practice*. Boston: Blackwell Scientific Publishing, pp. 353–367.

Carefoote, R. (1994). Total quality management implementation in home care agencies: Common questions and answers. *The Journal of Nursing Administration* 24 (10): 31–37.

Fitzpatrick, M. J. (1994). Performance improvement through quality improvement teamwork. *The Journal of Nursing Administration* 24 (12): 20–27.

Goode, C. J. (1995). Evaluating research-based nursing practice. *Nursing Clinics of North America* 30 (3): 421–428.

Greeneich, D. (1993). The link between new and returning business and quality of care: patient satisfaction. *Advances in Nursing Science* 16 (1): 62–72.

Jackson, J., C. P. Morgan, and J.G.P. Paolilla (1986). *Organizational Theory*. New York: Prentice-Hall Inc.

Lawton, B. R. (1993). The American roots of Deming and quality. In J. Eisenach and S. Hanser, eds., *Readings in Renewing American Civilization*. New York: McGraw-Hill.

Ludwig-Beymer, P., C. J. Ryan, N. J. Johnson, K. A. Hennessy, M. C. Gattuso, R. Epson, and K. T. Czurylos (1993). Using patient perceptions to improve quality of care. *Journal of Nursing Care Quality* 7 (2): 42–51.

Megel, M. E. and M.E.B Elrod (1993). Ethical and interpersonal conflicts experienced by nursing QA/QI professionals: Justice or care. *The Journal of Nursing Administration* 7 (4): 6–8.

Price, P. J. (1993). Parents' perceptions of the meaning of quality nursing care. *Advances in Nursing Science* 16 (1): 33–41.

Scott, W. R. (1981). *Organizations: Rational, Natural, and Open Systems.* New York: Prentice Hall Inc.

Sherman J. J. and M. A. Malkmus (1994). Integrating QA and TQM/QI. *The Journal of Nursing Administration* 24 (3): 37–41.

Shiber, S. and E. Larson (1991). Evaluation of the quality of caring: Structure, process, and outcome. *Holistic Nursing Practice* 5 (3): 57–66.

Thurston, N. E., L.A. Watson, and M. A. Reimer (1993). Research or quality improvement: Making the decision. *The Journal of Nursing Administration* 23 (7, 8): 41–49.

CHAPTER ELEVEN

The Organization and Practice of Nursing

This chapter will examine the practice and organization of nursing. It covers Benner's (1984) taxonomy of nurse practice, and some considerations of how to organize the health care system so as to enhance caring nursing practice.

Watson (1990) wrote about the failure of the patriarchy. She says that it is time to look at structural problems in the health care system to create environments where caring, healing, and the health work of nurses can exist. In the past, the work of women and nurses has been invisible, but a new paradigm is arising where caring and women's work can be identified and appreciated. The current model for health care and for our society has been the patriarchy, which elevates men and logic as primary forces. Watson asks if caring is something to fear because it can threaten human power, oppose control and domination, and make one vulnerable to human dilemmas, reminding us that we are all equally human and in need of caring. "The basis of the present condition of health care policy, politics, and practice and our present lack of caring consciousness and wider vision, are the results of a failure of our morality which demands a revolution of consciousness" (p. 63). Watson wants to see a movement away from the failed patriarchy toward a caring morality. Where the patriarchy was linear and pitted person against person and nation against nation, caring can contribute to the health and healing of individuals and nations. She notes that, if we constantly have to justify and defend our caring (as we often do in health care), it hardens our compassion and represses our emotions. If caring is to be sustained, those who care must be strong and courageous. The current morality that guides our health care policy is out of touch with the astonishing theoretical, philosophical, and scientific thinking that is transforming a new view of reality described repeatedly in this book. Watson asks, "Could it be that nursing's 'Invisible' caring is 'shadow matter' that fills in the void, offers a counterpoint for the chaotic forces in the universe?" (p. 65). She sees nursing as having a great responsibility in introducing the new paradigm, which is undergirded by caring. The struggle is on between those who would leave the force of logic and power in charge, and the forces in our society who are ready to receive and participate in a caring paradigm. Nursing's responsibility is awesome—in patient care and also in creating a new society—and the nurses who will lead this movement are nursing administrators who have embraced the values of caring and will bravely move the philosophy of caring into the dominant place in health care systems and in society. Caring cannot be our own little secret that we practice when no one is watching, it must be our proud service of everyday life.

As we consider the greatness of the caring paradigm, we must, at the same time, be realistic about where nursing is now and what nurses' work is really like. We must start by understanding real-life nurses, as did Benner (1984) in *From Novice to Expert*. In this book Benner reports on her study of nurses at various points in their careers. She found great differences in the nurses, which she classified as:

1. Novice: The rule-governed behavior typical of the novice is extremely limited. These new nurses (or ones who get stuck in this stage) have no experience to guide their work. They need rules to tell them how to behave in various situations. It reminds me of when I was a clinical teacher and went with a student for her first catheterization. She was so focused on the task she was just learning that she could give no attention to the patient. Most new nurses are

like this, and then they learn to move on in most cases (if not, you need to move them along).

2. Advanced Beginner: This nurse can demonstrate marginally acceptable performance including seeing the overall characteristics of the patient. They still require rules and procedure books to help them perform, and they need help in setting priorities. Where the novice nurse cannot function out of the student role, some advanced beginners can get by as new graduates with a preceptor to help them.

3. Competent: This category is typified by the nurse who has been on the job in the same or similar situations for two or three years. These nurses begin to see their actions in terms of long-term goals or plans, but lack the speed and flexibility of proficient nurses. Some nurses never get beyond this stage. We must ask ourselves if it is OK for us to have nurses at this level. Practically speaking, we could not run our health care systems without them. They are the middle-of-the-road workers who get the job done, but without any fanfare about it.

4. Proficient: These nurses understand situations as wholes because they perceive their meaning in terms of long-term goals. Decision making is easier, and they understand enough so that they do not have to consider every option. They are able to home in on an accurate region of the problem. These nurses are plentiful in health care settings. They will do well when left alone to do a full job proficiently.

5. Expert: These nurses no longer rely on an analytic principle to connect their understanding of the situation to an appropriate action. They have an intuitive understanding of situations, and zero in on the accurate region of the problem without wasteful consideration of unfruitful alternative diagnoses and solutions. The big advantage of expert nurses is that they operate from a deep understanding of the total situation. Experts dare to have hunches that can lead to early identification of problems (pp. 20–28).

Benner says that clinical knowledge is gained over time and that the nurses themselves are often unaware of their gains. One of the problems of expert nurses is that they typically give cryptic instructions that make sense only if the person hearing them has a deep understanding of the situation. Thus, it is frustrating and sometimes wasteful to have expert nurses trying to teach novice nurses. It is not possible to recapture from the experts the formal steps they go through to reach conclusions, because they do not build up their conclusions element by element. Rather, they grasp the whole of situations and know more than they can tell. Their knowledge is embedded in perceptions rather than identifiable facts. Benner believes that nurses can create healing climates by mobilizing hope, finding understanding of the situation, and assisting the patient in using social, emotional, and spiritual resources.

Benner's work has had an enormous impact on nursing and particularly nursing education. I think we need to look at the stages and ask what they mean to nursing and to caring. One of the problems a nursing administrator has is that of how to motivate nurses to do their best work. Perhaps Benner's description makes it easier to understand why all the nurses do not perform perfectly like we want them to. To me, understanding that there are different levels of nursing makes me more tolerant of nursing as a whole. When you become a nursing administrator, you don't want to hear about nurses who make mistakes or don't perform well all the time. When you begin to hear about things nurses do wrong or fail to do, you wonder why. We want all the nurses to be the expert practitioners we know or perhaps are. We want every nurse to long for primary nursing or case management, and we don't understand when there is no enthusiasm for programs that supposedly will benefit them, like career ladders or self-governance. There are always some nurses who want to be a part of all good projects, but we can't get other nurses out of their ruts. When I was first a nurse administrator, I was very frustrated about this. With time, I came to realize that nurse performance is like the bell-shaped curve—there are 10 percent or so that are the movers and shakers, another 10 percent or so that do not ever want to do anything, and the vast majority in the middle that can be influenced either way. I learned to appreciate all kinds of nurses as I realized that if they were all movers and shakers, it would be unmanageable. Likewise, if they were all willing to do nothing, we would have a very stagnant nursing division. We decided to let the movers and shakers forge ahead with projects, ignored the do-nothings, and spent a great deal of time on the vast majority that were the in-betweeners. By doing so, we were able to improve the practice of the majority of nurses, keep the movers and shakers moving, and deal with the nonperformers by discipline. One day a nurse told me, "I don't want to be a gung-ho nurse at this time in my life. I want to come to work, do a good job, and go home to my family." As I contemplated on this, I realized that I had been the same way when I had young children: I was mostly interested in my home life at that time in my life. And I realized that the bulk of nurses want to practice this way. That is why there is resistance to change and lack of enthusiasm to lead new programs. But our hospital could not operate without these nurses, who were probably proficient on Benner's scale. So, we gently nudged everyone forward until change didn't seem so bad and there was a lot of pride in their work for the majority of our nurses. We learned how to run things more smoothly, and the nurses learned that we would use their talents appropriately. Our nurses decided that they did not want a career ladder, and we found they worked harder and better if they felt we were listening. We spent one and a half years working on the career ladder and then threw it out when the nurses voted not to have it.

I have always been intrigued by the way nurses do their work. Before I became an administrator, I had been a staff nurse for twelve years, and I was not going to let go of the staff nurse role. I remembered a time when I had tried to become active in a staff nurse committee and immediately got in trouble with nursing administration. It was a shocking and very painful experience. I even contemplated leaving nursing. Well, I did not quit or totally stop getting into trouble, but I reached a conclusion: that taking care of patients was the mission of the hospital and the mission of my life's work, no matter what my role. That formed many of my opinions and actions for all my years in administration. The number-one criteria for what I did was its effect on patient care. I believed that my job was to set up systems that would allow clinical nurses to take optimal care of patients. I became interested in how nurses approached their work.

Botteroff and Morse (1994) studied the patterns of nurses' work. They focused on the nurse-patient interaction as the unit of study. They found five types of touch that nurses used with patients. They were comforting touch, connecting touch, working touch, orienting touch, and social touch. They also identified four types of attending: 1. Doing more (the nurse did something beyond what was required of them. It was characterized by concerned acknowledgment of the patient's concerns and systems, and frequently associated with patient distress or discomfort); 2. Doing for (the nurse was primarily occupied in responding to patient requests that were not treatment related. These nurses were trying to be more personable and friendly by doing little things for the patient); 3. Doing with (the nurse focused equally on the task and patient—showed a willingness to work with patient); 4. Doing tasks (the nurse was focused on equipment, treatment, and getting the work done. Patient comments were sometimes ignored because the nurse was so focused on the task).

This was of interest to me because it helped me understand what happens at the bedside. When I became an administrator, our system was functional nursing. It seemed to me that what that system did was to make the nurses more aware of their tasks than their patients (as in Bottorff and Morse's fourth type of attending). I was supervising some students before I became an administrator, and one day a student came to get me because she thought there was "something wrong" with one of her patients. Although the student had a nurse who she was supposedly working with, I went with her to see the patient. What I found was a patient in fulminating pulmonary edema. After we quickly got help and moved the patient to CCU, I reflected on how that could happen in this "top-notch" hospital. When I questioned the staff, the medicine nurse said she had seen how sick he was, but she had never seen him before and thought his condition might always be that way. To make a long story short, the rest of the staff said pretty much the same thing. As it turned out, no one had seen the patient twice except the student. Shortly after, I found a little article in a journal about the intellectual work of nursing. It said that tasks can be done without giving the patient nursing care. Functional and team methods of assignments make it difficult for a nurse to perform the intelligent work of nursing. The essence of nursing is the synthesis of data, and that can take place only if the nurse gathers the data and interprets its importance in the whole situation. It takes intelligence, time for reflection, and repeated experiences with the patient before the nurse can understand the whole situation the patient is in. That bit of advice has stayed with me. We have already discussed the changing nursing care delivery systems, many of which will once again take the nurse away from the patients and into supervising and paper functions. We have discussed the need for the nurse to feel she has done a "whole task" by providing all the care for one patient, but I guess I feel a need to reiterate these concerns in this section about the work of nursing. New systems must put the nurse closer to the patient, not further away. I was recently in a hospital where there were eight nurses to take care of sixteen critically ill patients. The problem was that only four of the nurses were giving the patient care; the rest were managers and nurse-specialists. So, of all the money allocated for nursing, only half of it was being spent on patient care. I see this as a problem, but it is typical of our high administrative costs in American health care. When I first started in administration, the situation was similar. We had charge nurses, medication nurses, team leaders, and ward secretaries. When we went to primary nursing, we did not have to add staff; we just reallocated all the nurses to doing patient care.

A physician, Tom Shragg, wrote in *The American Nurse* (1995) that most hospitals' plan for the future seems to be that of a CPA—one which returns us to an industrial model. He sees hospitals analyzing nurses' work into tasks that can be accomplished by cheaper providers. His example is of nurses giving a bath. Perhaps an undereducated nurse assistant can give the bath, but when an RN gives a bath, he/she can examine the patient's skin, nutrition, IV sites, bruises, drug reactions, and even the emotional state of the patient who is trembling and tearful. Shragg emphasizes that, in the future, physicians, nurses, and patients must play a part in shaping the health care system. "The bottom line can't be just a monetary one—taking care of patients is not just like slapping together a car" (p. 7).

Edwards and Horn (1995) wrote that the delivery of nursing care in multiple arenas is jeopardized by the injudicious use of unlicensed personnel. These people are trained to fill minimum-wage positions, but are often placed in patient care situations that require professional judgment, putting patients at risk. Edwards and Horn are concerned that health care is a "growth industry" concentrating on business aspects and lacking understanding and appreciation of the human element of care. Nursing administrators increasingly must choose between "playing on the team" or unemployment, and physicians are also being pressured to do what is best for the organization, not the patient. Edwards and Horn cry for a call to arms for nurses and physicians together to get involved in the health care reform battle.

Himali (1995), writing for the *American Nurse* (the official publication of the American Nurses Association), said that there are dangerous trends in hospital staffing that could jeopardize the quality and safety of patient care. Hospitals are cutting the numbers of registered nurses and replacing them with cheaper, minimally skilled workers. "The ANA believes that only when the public realizes the connection between registered nurses and safe, quality nursing care will there be an outcry against the widespread restructuring that is replacing RNs—some with 20 and 30 years experience—with unlicensed assistive personnel (UAP) who often have less than a month's training" (p. 1). ANA believes that "every patient deserves a nurse" and is working on a report card that would allow patients to evaluate nursing care.

During a recent hospitalization, the nurse executive visited me and asked me if my nursing care had been good. I guess I had been given just enough pain medication to be honest. I told her that the nurses were the best, but that I didn't see them much—that all my care was done by nurses' aides. I told her that they were perfectly nice people, but that they just did tasks, often two aids at a time, and often speaking to each other but not to me. I was really concerned one night when I was feeling bad, because I didn't know if I even had a nurse. All of my essential needs were met, I guess, but I didn't feel cared for. I think that is exactly what was missing—caring! The nurses' aids could do the functions, but they could not care in the way a nurse can. It is our commitment and our essence.

In a recent conversation with a nurse manager, he told me that their unlicensed workers were doing OK because they were nursing students. He said that he wondered, though, when he worked with them one day and found that they were talking to and teaching the patients while he (the nursing manager) was emptying urinals. Nursing always has a good plan for new systems, but when you take professional nurses away from the patients, you deny the patients what they need most—caring.

Now, I know that this is real old-fashioned thinking, and I know we must be more cost conscious, but to me, taking the nurses away from the bedside is the most cost unconscionable thing to do. Administrators (even some nursing administrators) do not understand the true costs of nurses' aids. They must be trained, they call in sick, they make mistakes, and they take up a lot of nurses' time getting their assignments and then reporting back what they did. And the work they do with patients falls short of the caring the patient needs and expects. The nurse's job becomes taking care of aids and the desk, not the patients. I feel certain that this return to an old system that did not work the first time will be unsuccessful again.

There are many studies that have documented that the costs of primary nursing and even all RN staffs were not more costly, and the patient and nurses were happier. I am even more concerned about using nurses' aids in today's hospital environment, where all the patients are too sick to be cared for by nonprofessionals. Administrators do not understand that, when nurses are giving baths or changing beds, they have an opportunity to observe and interact with the patient. Nursing is more than a list of tasks that we dole out to the cheapest provider. My philosophy is to hire non-nurses to do all the work *outside* the patients' rooms. There is plenty of waste in nurses' time because of inadequate support systems. Give that work to someone else, and leave the patient's care to the professional nurses. When nurses are *with* patients, they can be caring. If they are not, what is left of the caring we espouse as the essence of nursing? Let the nurse spend maximum time with patients so that healing relationships can develop and caring can grow. When patients have nurses to confide in and trust, they get well quicker and leave with glowing accounts of their hospital stay.

I know that nurse administrators are being pushed and sometimes ordered to reduce the case mix (RNs to aids), and I know there are some cases where innovative systems can maintain nurses at the bedside. But nurse administrators of today and tomorrow need to think about the caring in the systems, not just the costs. In my earlier example, a patient nearly died with good nurses all around that were in a bad system. Administrators need to hear of the bad instances when the system doesn't work, and nurse administrators must watch carefully for patients' less-satisfied responses about their nursing care. We need to be alert when other departments begin complaining that nursing isn't doing its job, and we must listen carefully for grumblings of dissatisfaction among the nursing staff.

Another new nursing care delivery system that has taken hold is case management. In some cases it may be the best route to go. If this is a way to connect patients and nurses for long-term relationships, it may greatly enhance the caring the patient receives. But if it means that nurse case managers will know the patients by making rounds like doctors, it will not contain the same closeness that occurs when the nurse is with the patient all day or night. Case management is creating exiting new jobs for nurses, but I hope we do case management in a way that does not diminish the bedside nurse. Nurses should all have the opportunity to provide caring to patients.

Curtin (1986) wrote an editorial titled, "Who says lean must be mean?" She says that if physicians produce "products," they might be called medical diagnoses. The federal government has, for their product, DRGs. But hospitals neither diagnose nor prescribe, and the hospital's "product" is *patient care*. She emphasizes that the American Hospital Association has said that 90 percent of patient care is delivered by nurses. At the same time, nursing takes up only 30 percent of the hospital's costs. Curtin thinks it is quite a bargain to get 90 percent of the product with 30 percent of your costs.

You may recall that the Pew Fetzer Report focused attention on relationship-centered care. Its authors reported that the national debate over health care reform focuses on access and financing and much less on the actual dynamics or quality of care. Relationships between patients and practitioners are the medium of exchange for all forms of information, feelings, and concerns, and are frequently the most therapeutic aspect of the health care encounter. Health is a sense of coherence (that is, a sense that life is comprehensible, manageable, and meaningful) and an ability to function in the face of changes in oneself and his/her relationships with the environment. Since supportive relationships are one of the factors promoting healing, the relationship between healer and patient is of utmost importance. The practitioners' relationship with their patients and the patients' communities are a vehicle for putting into action a paradigm of health that integrates caring, healing, and community. In order to maintain caring/healing relationships with patients, the practitioner needs knowledge and skills, respect for the patients' dignity, acceptance and compassionate responses, and attention to his/her own distress and the patient's pain. The practitioner must value the patients' own power and self-healing.

These are powerful words about patient care. They support a caring response in all aspects of patient care. They also bring attention to the importance of nurses' work. It is important to note that the Pew Fetzer Report came from a multidisciplinary group including non-care-providers. I often think that we in nursing "preach to the converted" in that we keep our ideas within nursing. I wish this book would be read by non-nurses too, so that they could see our passionate desire to practice caring with our patients.

Maeve (1994) described the "carrier bag" theory of nursing practice. She iterates that nursing's identity lies in relationships—in relationships *between* patients and their physicians, the hospital system, bureaucrats, and other health care personnel, as well as between family, friends, and the community. We literally "carry" the patient's interests to all parts of their health care experience. Nursing can be seen as a web of connections, and the ordeal of the in-between stance is a reality that we fail to adequately prepare nurses for. She writes:

> The carrier bag theory of nursing is about the everyday practice of bedside nursing. It is about bedside nurses who continue the oral and experiential tradition that has kept nursing alive since the dawn of time through the sharing of experiences directly or through the recounting of them in stories and narratives. Further, the carrier bag theory of nursing practice depends on individual nurses' and individual patients' experiences of care to know and define excellence in practice.
>
> (pp. 20–21)

This is an unusual way to look at nursing, but, I dare say, many nurses have experienced feeling like a carrier bag at their work setting.

Now that we have considered nurses' work, let us turn our attention to how to manage in a nursing environment. McCloskey (1989) wrote about requirements for job contentment. She said that "it is generally believed that the restructuring of the work setting to increase the decision-making power of staff nurses is the key to nurse recruitment and retention" (p. 140). Another concept that she sees reemerging is that of caring, which some may see as at odds with the concept of autonomy. I think of them as synonymous. While feeling a strong desire for autonomy, the nurse's job is to care, and yet they also need to care for themselves. And an important source of support for nurses comes from their nurse peers. McCloskey surveyed 320 nurses about autonomy and social integration. She found that both autonomy and social integration are important for nurses. Even if nurses have one or the other, they remain relatively satisfied and motivated, but if both are low, nurses are less satisfied, have less commitment and motivation, and have less intent to remain on the job. The nurses most affected by this are those who are most experienced and those with more education. She concludes that what nurses want is autonomy with connectedness.

This study was done when there was a perceived nursing shortage. Now we have an abundance of nurses, since many organizations are replacing nurses with nurses' aids. It is still an important study, though, if we believe in the organizational theorists who see employee satisfaction as crucial to the operation of successful businesses. I think, in the 1990s, nurses crave autonomy and social belonging more than ever. As nurse administrators plan for the future, we can count on the need to keep nurses satisfied by providing some sort of self-governance and peer group connection. In one hospital I know, each unit is given one workshop day a year at a site away from the hospital (they have to either use a vacation day or an unpaid day off, so its not really given to them; any employee can decide not to come, but that is rare). They have educational material and an update from administration, but they also have fun time planned so that they can feel more cohesive as a group. It has been a very healthy experience for most nurses on the involved units.

As nurses find ways to support themselves in their practice, it is up to nursing administration to help staff feel in control in their patient care setting. Wolf, Boland, and Aukerman (1994) wrote about a transformational model for nursing practice. They acknowledge the existing paradigm shifts, like most of our writers, and define the need for a different model of nursing practice in the future. They say that nursing's practice must evolve from a needs-based system to a resource-sensitive one. While nurses have been socialized to meet all of a patient's needs, these authors contend that patients do not expect all of their health care needs to be met: only those they consider to be important. These authors say that as resources become more limited, nurses must negotiate with patients to determine the critical needs and plan for the most effective use of resources to meet those needs. In the future, they say, achieving quality must be accomplished through critical thinking focused on the unique needs of each patient, coupled with creative approaches for meeting these needs.

While I appreciate the reality of scarce resources, I am not sure that I agree that patients don't want all their needs met. The people I talk with who have been hospitalized complain loudly about the lack of nursing care. They say that a $2,000 a day bill ought to mean that their needs are met. I think patients will understand if the nurses have a bad shift, but for the hospitalization as a whole, they want the kind of care that meets their needs. I believe that word will quickly get out if a hospital is chronically understaffed in nursing. I agree with Mallison (1985) that the hospital winners will compete by delivering a product that supplies superior value to customers, rather than one that costs less. As the tide of health care continues to roll, nursing care is its staple, and scrimping on the staple is short-sighted. We can contain costs to a certain level, and then the morale of the patient and the nurse will fall apart.

Recently, I was discussing nursing administration with a vice-president for nursing, and she reminded me that there is a critical mass where situations feed on themselves. This can be a positive or a negative thing. If new programs and increased autonomy excite the nurses who are the go-getters, their enthusiasm often spreads to the whole staff, and the workplace becomes a happy and productive place. Conversely, if the nurses consistently feel overworked and unable to meet patients' needs, the negative emotions can spread throughout the staff and even to the patients. The good part of working with new paradigms that are resource-driven is that the nurses may be able to make adjustments in their own expectations so that they can feel better about their work. But, we must be very cautious in seeing that the expectations of the patients are the same as those of the nurses. If the two are not congruent, nurse administrators must be very clear about what is happening at the patient level and remind administration that the product is patient care.

Manthey (1990) reminds us that relationships determine staff morale, and that is the single most vital determinant of patient care quality. She says that today's nurse manager is the one who manages the staff who manage the care. Manthey says that morale is a function of how the staff members treat one another, not how others treat them. She denounces "Mama Management" and advocates giving moral support from the sidelines, but refusing to take over. By letting nurses go, they can become confident and autonomous in their practice and develop into happy, competent staffs.

Prescott and Dennis (1985) wrote about power in hospital nursing departments. They believe that nurses should be meaningfully involved in the running of hospitals. They did a study to see if nurses felt that they had power in the hospital. Fifty-three percent of staff nurses felt they could influence policies and thirty percent said they had no input into policies. The authors said it was clear that staff nurses as a group were not the final source of authority for nursing care policies. They had only a

A Caring Approach in Nursing Administration

vague knowledge of how policies were enacted in their organizations. They perceived an institutional lockstep of lengthy procedures for enacting policies, and they were not willing to tolerate the system. The overall tone of the staff nurses' responses reflected a lack of power awareness and ineffective use of expertise as a source of power. The supervisors and nurse administrators felt that the nurses had power, but the nurses themselves did not perceive it. Forty-four percent of the nurses described relationships with nursing administration as distant.

Porter-O'Grady (1986) describes workers' fundamental needs. They are: 1. autonomy or control over their work behavior; 2. completion or achievement of a whole task; and 3. a level of interpersonal contacts within the work activities themselves. We need to find ways of correlating the needs of the institution and nurses so that the purposes of both can be fulfilled. Participation for nurses must be found in setting goals, making decisions by choosing from among alternative courses of action, solving problems through definition of issues, generation of altered courses of action, and making changes in the organization.

Nursing departments have put enormous energy into developing participative management and self- or shared-governance programs in the last decade. Havens (1994) studied hospitals to see if nurses were indeed feeling more input into decisions in their hospitals. Findings suggested that models for professional governance had not been implemented on a wide-spread basis by 1990. Staff nurses saw themselves as being able only to give input into decisions, and that their input may or may not be acted on. A national survey of nurse executives in the late 1980s suggested that shared governance was the buzzword and was projected to be implemented by 1992. However, on most units in this 1994 study, governance was not shared. Havens says that these findings suggest a degree of conceptual confusion regarding the definition of shared governance in nursing. She suggests that staff nurses, managers, and administrators must work together to create and maintain environments and structures that support professional governance for health care organizations.

My own experience is that hospitals that were advocating shared governance in the 1980s have found it very difficult to maintain these systems. In one hospital I know of, when it came time for tough decisions (cutting staff), the nurse administration backtracked from their governance model, and the decisions came down from nursing administration with no consultation with staff. It is very difficult to maintain participative models when the decisions you are asked to make will negatively affect the participants. As health care as a whole recoils from participative decision making to a stronger bureaucracy, it is hard for nursing not to do the same. It is hard to ask nurses to care for more and sicker patients, and then tell them they have no input into decisions. But, if we want to maintain caring in our patient care environmental, nurses must be respected and treated like the professionals they are. We must continue to work on participative or shared-governance-type models.

Rost (1994) wrote about a new conception of management. He argues that the common wisdom is that leadership is indefinable, that leaders are all about doing great things that help make the world go around, and that they do things that help all people to live the good life. There also is common wisdom that followers are to do "followership"— do the leader's wishes, and be passive, subordinate, submissive, unintelligent, unproductive, not in control of their lives, and thus needing leaders to show them the way. Rost defines this as the industrial paradigm of leadership, which he sees as no longer acceptable. Instead, he advocates a postindustrial paradigm of leadership. Rost says that (as we have read over and over) paradigm shifts occur during tumultuous times when basic assumptions about life, living, organizations, societies, professions, and academic disciplines are questioned and transformed. He believes that we are now experiencing paradigm shifts in medicine, nursing, health care delivery systems, education, politics, global-mindedness, environmental care, spirituality, and organizations and leadership that all will bring us into the postindustrial era of the twenty-first century.

In the new paradigm, leadership is an influence relationship among leaders and "collaborators" (his new word for followership) who intend real changes that reflect their mutual purposes. He defines four elements of leadership that must all be present to be called leadership: 1. both leaders and collaborators are involved in the relationship; 2. they use only noncoercive influence strategies in that relationship; 3. they intend real (significant) changes; and 4. they make sure that the changes reflect the mutual purposes of collaborators and leaders. The postindustrial megaparadigm will focus on collaboration, active participation, common good, pluralism, client orientation, and consensus building. Collaborators do not do followership: they do leadership. In the new paradigm, leadership

A Caring Approach in Nursing Administration

is not about governance or management/administration. It is about change, and management/administration is about the day-to-day activities that go into operating a group, organization, and society. The new paradigm will include an entire constellation of beliefs, values, and techniques that will lead us into the twenty-first century. Rost sees leadership as an episodic affair, not what people in management or administration do all day, but an episodic process in which leaders and collaborators form a relationship to change a group, organization, or society. We will need professionals, academics, leaders, and collaborators working together in a relationship to institute real, mutually agreeable changes in our whole constellation of beliefs, values, and techniques to construct a new reality.

The reason I include Rost's work in this chapter is that I think it points to the way nursing administrators must act in the future. We have seen dozens of references about changing paradigms and the need for management/administration to change direction. Nowhere is the change needed more than in nursing. In the past, it may have been adequate for nursing leaders to tell staff nurses what to do. But, the leaders now have no way to keep up with enough clinical knowledge to tell staff what to do. The best we can hope for is that nurses at all levels work together to direct nursing's future.

Whereas Rost calls old followers collaborators, I call them colleagues. I believe we will still need leaders (perhaps with a different name) to help the systems roll along, but they should not be seen as any more important than clinical nurses. The real work comes from clinical nurses, and administrators who make sure the system supports the clinicians. The product is patient care, not the dollars generated by the organization. Success is happy, well-cared-for patients, not happy, well-cared-for administrators.

I believe that a health care organization has many clients, including doctors (although more and more of them are becoming employees), suppliers (I agree with Deming that relationships with suppliers should be cultivated so that supplies are useful and of reasonable cost, which is more likely to occur if there is an ongoing relationship with the supplier), employees (I believe that happy employees are more likely to do a good job if they feel valued by the organization), patients and their families (the most important clients of all), professionals (which I see as different than employees), and the community and society. In a way, I think even the administrators are clients, as the organization is their source of income and job satisfaction. Viewing all these people as clients is important because it clarifies the organization as a group of people interacting for their own and others' good. It means that the most important part of the organization is how the people interact, and that is where caring comes in.

To me, the new paradigm for leadership and following is simply *caring!* I do have some reservations about whether or not health care administrators (non-nursing) have come to the place where they understand or use the new paradigm of thinking, and in particular, a caring paradigm. This is because of some of the information presented earlier about bureaucracies and economic values. I think many of them are in a survival mode, and all they can attend to is dollars. But I also believe that nursing administrators are increasingly influencing their administrations, and this will be a real key to moving all health care administrators toward a caring paradigm.

Scott (1982) defines three types of organizational models for managing professionals. The first type is the autonomous professional organization, where organizational officials delegate to the professional group responsibility for defining and implementing the goals, for setting up performance standards, and for seeing to it that standards are maintained. This is the model that physicians have operated in for many years. This organizational form works well when work is regarded as unusually complex, uncertain, and of great social importance. The professional body is given the responsibility of controlling and evaluating themselves as it is difficult for anyone who does not have their knowledge base to evaluate their work. There is a sharp demarcation between the professional and administrative zones of control, and the professional comes to use the organization without being supervised by the organization.

The second type of organizational model is the heteronomous organization, where professionals are clearly subordinated to the administrative structure. This system has grown with the increasing power of hospital administrators and medical managers within hospitals. Nurses were used as an example of professionals in this type of organization. The amount of autonomy granted the professionals is somewhat circumscribed. Participants in these settings are more constrained by administrative controls and subject to routine supervision. The leaders of the professionals are responsible to the organization more than to the professionals. This model revolves around an organizational hierarchy that is strong and controlling. Scott says that physicians are moving in the direction of the heteronomous model as they become more and more enmeshed in hospital affairs. The power shifts away from the individual physicians to organizational arrangements supporting a well-defined division of labor. More and more physicians are becoming employed by health care organizations, and peer review organizations are set up to review the work of physicians. One problem with this type of organization is that it may disrupt the relationship between patient and practitioner with less attention to patient concerns and more attention to the problems of the organization. The presumption is that those designing the control system know better than the professionals about what types of decisions and behaviors are necessary or preferred. Heteronomous organizations exhibit a relatively high proportion of administrators and supervisors. In general, the more complex the work and the higher the qualifications of workers, the larger and more elaborate the hierarchy. The increase in supervisors signifies not increased closeness of supervision but an attempt to improve the transmission of information and the decision-making capacity of the organization. Some physicians are most unhappy about the move to the heteronomous organizational model. "Professionals see themselves as moral, autonomous actors, responsible and accountable for their own decisions, hence, needing to resist all efforts to regulate their actions. They emphasize the critical importance of decision making on a case by case basis and resist the notion that there are abstract or all-purpose formulas adequate to regulate their work" (Scott 1982, p. 56).

The third kind of organization examined by Scott is called the conjoint professional organization. This model is more the author's ideas rather than an extant model. In this type of organization, professional participants and administrators are roughly equal in the power that they command and in the importance of their functions. They coexist in a state of interdependence and mutual influence. Scott recognizes that, in this type of organization, conflict will be increased as people learn to work with each other rather than for one another. This model allows the integration of physicians into the organizational setting.

This article was primarily written from a physician's point of view, but I think it is extremely important as we consider the organizational model that is best for nursing. It helps me see that the model we are currently in is a mixture of these models, and that we need to consider carefully where we want nursing to be in relation to the organizations we work in. As nurses have become more autonomous and independent, they want less hierarchy to restrain them. As the physicians move more into an organizational model where they lose some autonomy, nurses are trying to shake off the heavy-handed organizational structure. I hope we can move nurses to the conjoint or even the autonomous organizational model where they clearly see the patient as their primary responsibility, not the organization. Shared or self-governance models would increase the staff's autonomy, but it seems that these models have had very limited success. The important element of any new governance structure should be to increase the caring relationship with patients, not their dependence on the organizational structures.

In defining systems for the work of nursing, a popular trend is the "patient-centered" model. This seems a little hollow when nursing staffs are being cut, but it is another buzzword or initiative. Boston (1995) writes that in a recent survey focusing on trends in patient-centered projects, nearly one-half of the responding organizations reported major work redesign projects either underway or being planned. This author notes that it is one thing to redesign a delivery system model and quite another to actually transform the core work, philosophy, or culture so that patient-focused care is internalized and maximized by all employees throughout the organization. It certainly is hopeful, though, that so many organizations are recognizing patients' needs and desires. I remember when it was a fad to bring in consultants to teach staff how to be nice to customers, like McDonalds and Walmart do. Our nurses were somewhat offended at the inference that they needed training in relating to patients, but in the end they said they learned a little and hoped it would make the organization as a whole more patient-oriented. If an organization decides it wants to be more patient-centered, that is *great*. It should translate to adequate numbers of nurses and proper nursing models that create what we are all about—caring! Because, if you ask patients what the most important thing was in their hospitalization, they will almost always say, "THE NURSES."

This chapter has concentrated on the organization of the work of nurses. It has broad implications for nursing administrators as it begins to define the work of those persons who occupy such positions. I would say at this point, that what we have learned about nursing and caring pretty much deflates the possible success of authoritative nurse administrators in this day and age. The organizations we have described need facilitators and intuitive leaders who help others to reach their potential. Modern-day health care organizations cry out for caring in the actions of their leaders and their staffs. I hope they find that in nursing and nursing administration.

References

Benner, P. (1984). *From Novice to Expert.* Menlo Park, CA: Addison-Wesley.

Boston, C. (1995). Cultural transformation. *The Journal of Nursing Administration* 25 (1): 19–20.

Botteroff, J. N., and J. M. Morse, (1994). Identifying types of attending: Patterns of nurses' work. *Image: Journal of Nursing Scholarship* 26 (1): 53–60.

Curtin, L. L. (1986). Who says lean must be mean. *Nursing Management* 17 (1): 7–8.

Edwards, D. S. and P. A. Horn (1995). War on many fronts. Troubling trends in health care delivery. *The Journal of Nursing Administration* 25 (5): 5–7.

Havens, D. C. (1994). Is shared governance being shared? *The Journal of Nursing Administration* 24 (6): 59–64.

Himali, U. (1995). ANA sounds alarm about unsafe staffing levels: PR campaign sheds light on RN replacement trends. *The American Nurse* (March): 1, 12, 14, 16, 17.

Maeve, K. M. (1994). The carrier bag theory of nursing practice, *Advances in Nursing Science* 16 (4): 9–22.

Mallison, M. B. (1985). Passionate about excellence. *American Journal of Nursing* (June): 635.

Manthey, M. (1990). From "mama management" to team spirit. *Nursing Management* 21 (1): 20–21.

McCloskey, J. C. (1989). Two requirements for job contentment: Autonomy and social integration. *Image: Scholarship of Nursing Scholarship* 22 (3): 140–142.

Porter-O'Grady, T. (1986). *Creative Nursing Administration: Participative Management for the 21st Century.* Rockville, MD: Aspen Publications.

Prescott, P. A. and K.E. Dennis (1985). Power and powerlessness in hospital nursing department. *Journal of Professional Nursing* (Nov.–Dec.): 348–355.

Rost, J. C. (1994). Leadership: A new conception. *Holistic Nursing Practice* 9 (1): 1–8.

Scott, W. R. (1982). Managing professional work: Three models of control for health organization. *Health Services Research* 17 (3): 213–240.

Shragg, T. (1995). Where's the patient in the 'industrial model' of care? *The American Nurse* (June): p. 56.

Tresolini, C. P., and the Pew-Fetzer Task Force. (1994) *Health Professions Education and Relationship-Centered Care.* San Francisco, CA: Pew Health Professions Commission, 1994.

Watson, J. (1990). The moral failure of the patriachy. *Nursing Outlook* 38 (2): 62–66.

Wolf, G. A., S. Boland, and M. Aukerman (1994). A transformational model for the practice of professional nursing. *The Journal of Nursing Administration* 24 (4): 51–57, 24 (5): 38–46.

CHAPTER TWELVE

Practicing Caring
Nursing Administration

This last chapter will focus on the practice of nursing administration in a caring manner. The previous chapters have led us to this point by defining caring, introducing organizational and leadership theories that are compatible with caring, finding ethics and values that reinforce caring, wrestling with economic issues related to caring, and introducing research and effectiveness measures that help evaluate caring systems.

As we have discussed earlier, some authors do not see nurses as having much leadership potential. I, on the other hand, believe that most nurses have some foundational abilities that enhance their potential for leadership. These are:

1. *Interactive-relational skills.* Nurses, By the nature of their work, become experts in dealing with all kinds of people. This is one of the hardest things to teach students of management. Nurses can lead all kinds of people, encouraging them to be independent and successful, as we do with patients. We can deal with difficult people, and have expert communication skills. These are very important skills for managers.

2. *Patient care emphasis.* For nurses, consideration of patient care naturally comes first. We are the people who spend all of our time in the workplace meeting patient needs. Hospital managers who have done no patient care have a very difficult time imagining patient needs and considerations. Therefore, the decisions they make might very well make no sense at the bedside. The nurse who goes into management has a very important perspective to bring to the administrative table.

3. *Caring as foundational.* This book is dedicated to making nurses more aware of their caring mission. We have said that caring is the essence of nursing, and when a nurse goes into administration she takes caring as a basis of life along with her. This does not mean that we are just aware of caring as it relates to patient care; it refers to our approach to life. It can mean a great deal to an administration team to have a caring person as a part of the group. In management, there is often a lot of game playing and competition, and a caring member can make the environment more pleasant and more productive.

4. *Coordinating.* This is a very important skill for managers/administrators, and it is also hard to teach. Nurses coordinate every day as they work with other providers to get services to patients in an efficient and effective way. We are the masters of coordination in health care, and that is another skill that is very important in management.

5. *Holistic view.* Nurses are taught early on to see patients as holistic persons who have a families and worlds beyond the health care problems they may be experiencing. This helps nurse managers to develop a holistic view of the organization. We do not see problems as mechanical problems to be solved, but as problems with a complex environment that must be taken into consideration with people-oriented problems.

6. *Health promotion.* Nurses are taught to value health promotion, and it seems like the health care system is finely catching up to the importance of health care promotion in the ultimate health status of our population. We also know how to teach health promotion so that patients can accept it, and this skill will be very valuable as organizations set up systems of health promotion.

7. *Collegiality.* Nurses have learned that their jobs are very stressful, and that they need to have support systems to relieve the stress. We have learned to rely on each other and to value each other as colleagues. This makes it easier to enter an administrative group and encourage the group to be supportive of each other, not competitors.

8. *Working within a system.* Nurses have had to deal with "the system" for their whole careers. They understand when to make decisions on their own and when to ask for help from their supervisors. As we try to decentralize our organizations, it will be very important to know when to act, when to delegate, and when to ask for help. Nurses have much experience with making these calls, and can help other administrators to do the same.

I believe that these abilities are extremely important for potential nurse managers, and that present administrators should be aware of this and encourage appropriate nurses to go into management. In the past, nursing has often promoted its best clinicians, and this has, in some cases, been an extremely bad choice. Administrators may use these foundational abilities to judge which nurses show a propensity for management.

Blair (1976) wrote that, in the 1970s, there was a dearth of prepared nursing administrators. She says that, in the previous twenty-five years, the emphasis of graduate nursing programs had been focused on increasing the numbers of clinical nurse researchers, and that nursing administration had been ignored. Dr. Blair started a nursing administration program funded by the Kellogg Foundation with three assumptions: 1. successful nursing administration depends on an advanced knowledge of nursing; 2. nursing administration is committed to the attainment of broad health goals for society that are shared with other professions; and 3. successful nursing administration focuses on dynamic interchange within a system and between systems.

I was privileged to be a student in the second graduating class of Dr. Blair's program. We were very aware that we were in a test program. The university wasn't sure about the program, so we had to do both clinical and administration requirements. Probably the best part of the curriculum was that we took all our organization classes with the health care administration students. It was more than a little interesting. Most of the health care administration students had no clinical experience, yet there was a bias that they were somehow a little better than the nursing students. I remember one class when a health care administrator student asked a question, and the professor answered by saying something derogatory about administrators who walk through nursing units without saying anything to the staff. The student said, "What's wrong with that?" The nurses all groaned, and we never again felt inferior to the health administration students. It was a wonderful lesson for me, because I had always been frustrated by administrators who seemed to think they were too good to talk to the staff. Now I knew that, to some extent, they just didn't know any better.

By 1989, Blair and her nursing administration master's program were well thought of, and she wrote again of nursing administration. This time, she said that the major role for nurse executives was insuring excellence in all aspects of the organization's patient care program. She saw an expanded role and said that nurses in executive positions can no longer see themselves as concerned only with the nursing aspects of the organization. Blair saw nursing administration education as a synthesis of management knowledge and nursing knowledge whereby the two fields are integrated into a specific knowledge base. She wrote that:

> The nursing executive must use knowledge of caring acquired from a nursing perspective and knowledge from a business perspective to maintain a creative tension in the battle of things vs. people. Cost control cannot be allowed to displace care-giving personnel. . . . (the nurse administrator) must be able to make administrative decisions that promote the humanistic elements in patient care but protect the economic side of the enterprise.
>
> (1989, p. 9)

Now we will turn our attention to the administrators who are now in position, and we will examine how they are practicing and how they can integrate caring into their practice. In 1979, when I was a young administrator, I was asked to speak to a group of nursing administration professors about how to practice nursing administration. I organized my talk around two primary roles that I still believe are the key roles for the nursing administrators. One role is to be a leader of a profession, and the second is to be a facilitator in the health care organization. Now, I would modify those roles to be: 1. Leader of a caring profession, and 2. Facilitator of caring in a health care organization.

As the leader of a caring profession, the nurse administrator has an enormous job. Nurses need to have a leader who is listened to and who listens. This seems obvious enough, but it has always been the biggest problem for nursing administrators. Schoenhofer (1994) asks, "How are nurse executives portraying their distancing from the heart of nursing? How and why might nursing administrators move to reconnect with those persons, nurses and those they nurse, who look to them for ministry? What, for example, do nurse executives individually and collectively portray about distance from the heart of nursing when they seek professional identity and political alignment not with the nursing aspect of their role, but with the executive?" (p. 4).

Klakovich (1994) also wrote that front-line nurses feel abandoned by their nursing leaders, and that the feelings of abandonment have increased with the tendency to move the director of nursing to the position of vice-president for nursing or patient care services. As the nurse executive becomes less visible, the staff feels that they have left nursing to join the administrative elite. She asks, "How can nurses continue to care for their patients in a stressful environment that devalues clinical practice and abandons or alienates staff nurses?" (p. 43).

Sarosi and O'Conner (1993) suggest one method of keeping connected to staff nurses. Nursing rounds have traditionally been a way to keep in touch. However, they were often stressful and superficial. Nurses wondered what the nurse executive wanted to hear, and the nurse executive felt that she was imposing on the very busy staff nurses. Sarosi and O'Conner suggest the method of storytelling where six to eighteen participants gather in a quiet room with a facilitator who models a good story. The skilled storyteller tries to convey the magic of living stories and prepare the participants to tell their own stories about their experiences with patients. The key is in the listening. Sarosi and O'Conner say you need to "listen with your bones" in a state of intuitive listening. The elements of storytelling are: 1. story cue (why do I recall this story); 2. the shock cue (what triggered the insight, feeling, sensation that caused such a deep imprint on the memory); and 3. significance cue (what value or response or question about life is revealed in the story?). The nurse executives who tried the storytelling method found it to be more meaningful and enlightening than regular rounds. They reported feeling positive and energized by the storytelling.

When I was a nurse administrator, I made it a strong priority to stay connected to staff nurses, but it was very hard. I thought I was doing a pretty good job until a staff nurse said to me, "You used to be such a nice person when you were a staff nurse, what happened?" I was crushed. As I talked with my peers about it, I came to understand that putting on the title of nurse administrator automatically put up some walls. I saw myself as a nurse of nurses, but staff were not so sure any more. Then I had the opposite experience. I tried to be a representative administrator, so at an administration meeting, I said something about "the nurses think this . . ." One administrator asked me why I asked the nurses about things when my job was to tell the nurses what to do. It is a tightrope walk to stay connected to staff nurses and yet be an administrator. I believe nurses want and need leaders who will support nursing in an enthusiastic and sensitive manner. I think they also want nursing leaders that will hold their own in the board room and contribute to the organization as a whole. They want nursing administrators who have a strong belief system and a vision of nursing that the whole nursing division can believe in and work together to achieve. What they do *not* want is a nurse leader that has left nursing behind and can only see the organization's problems. They want a leader who loves caring and nursing and patient care and can take that view with them into the organizational arena.

As nurse executives take caring with them, they must enter the executive suite and translate that caring into organizational caring. Smith et al. (1994) wrote that the nurse executive, acting as a liaison and mediator between nursing staff and administration, is an essential member of the administrative team. She says that nurse executives must be flexible, action-oriented, have executive level business skills, and be experts on clinical affairs. Other desired qualities include credibility, trustworthiness, creativity, and willingness to change. They must also have a sense of caring, hope, optimism, and self-esteem.

The issue of the administrator being a clinical expert has a long and unsettled history. With clinical knowledge bursting out of its boundaries again and again, it is obviously impossible for the nursing administrator to be current in one area, let alone all areas of practice. I think staff nurses understand that reality and do not expect the nurse executive to step into a clinical situation and always be able to function. I know that, when I spent a shift on a unit to keep myself grounded in patient care, the nurses never let me do anything dangerous. They would tease me about not knowing things, but they seemed pleased to have me enter their world for a time. The issue is not so cut and dried with nursing shift supervisors or unit nurse managers. Nurses do expect them to be able to help in clinical situations. As nurse managers have been asked to do more and more management tasks, some staff nurses feel a lack of understanding from the nurse managers. The more managers, the more management work there is, and one more layer is seen as being out of touch with "real nursing." More space is perceived between the nurse executive and staff. Whatever the situation, it is the nurse executive's responsibility to find ways to stay in touch with staff nurses. This is the only way to continue to be a leader of a caring profession.

Stivers (1991) wrote that, despite the emergence of new theories, organizational and political leadership are still culturally masculine. Some feminists' approach is to adopt the mainstream definition and teach women to be tough, bold, etc. Another approach is to adopt the theory that women's unique qualities are significant and of value in their own right. This book has focused on the second alternative. Nurse administrators face the dilemma of female leadership in a particular way. As a nurse, the nurse administrator sees her objective as facilitating care and caring. Stivers says, "As an administrator, however, the nurse administrator is expected to answer a different mandate—one responsive to organizational needs, such as minimizing costs, deploying and using resources efficiently, inducing employees to put organizational goals ahead of their own, protecting organizational prerogatives, and maximizing the organization's control over its environment. These have traditionally been masculine concerns" (p. 49).

I see the situation as a little less conflicted. To me, putting caring first is not just better for the nurses—it is just as important to organizational success. Caring is the goal of all administrative affairs. Stivers says that the question becomes not "what mix of attention to caring and efficiency is in the patient's and society's best interests?" but rather "how much caring can we afford?" Nurse administrators may find that issue as striking at the heart of their professional identity. They have to retain caring as their profession's goal and find ways to make the rest of the organization understand what caring means to the whole organization.

In interviewing nurse administrators, Stivers found their biggest management problem was balancing care and economics (exactly what I found in 1989). The nursing administrators also were very concerned with their abilities to "see the big picture." The nurse administrators must be acknowledged as managers and as members of a women's profession. They face unique contradictions and the universal tension between health care quality and cost. Nurse administrators must both "be themselves" and practice with the knowledge of the "big picture" of their organization and beyond.

Miller (1989) writes about the role of a facilitator of caring in the organization as she describes a corporate view of nurse executive leadership. She stresses that nurse leaders are taking on roles that include policymaking, marketing, economics, and strategic planning. Nurses must be educated to understand organizational climates and the impact of corporate culture. They must create ways to maintain the caring perspective in a potentially uncaring organizational environment. Corporate responsibilities may take nurse executives away from the realities of bedside nursing, and the nurse executive must find committee structures or other mechanisms to keep in touch with nurses. Miller says that the success of the nursing department depends on the ability of the nurse executive to balance economic productivity and quality patient care. The nurse leaders must be caring to the nurses so that the nurses can be caring to the patients.

Klakovich (1994) wrote about connective leadership, a leadership model that connects individuals to their tasks and visions and to one another, to the immediate group and the larger network, inspiring others and instilling confidence. Connective leadership can be achieved when the nurse executive takes on departments other than nursing and works to integrate them into a high-performance patient care organization instead of a bunch of competing, separate departments. The connective leader excels at recognizing and nurturing strengths in others. They bring others into the leadership process and foster their ability to work synergistically. With this leadership strategy, there is the potential to provide a caring professional practice environment where everyone works toward the achievement of common goals.

While I write about the roles of the nurse executive as a leader of a caring profession and a facilitator of caring in the organization, McClure (1989) has written of two roles of nurse executives as those of care-giver and of integrator. She avers that nurse administrators make a unique contribution to the executive suite because they are more familiar with the product than most other administrators. She agrees that the role of the nurse administration is: 1. leader in a clinical discipline of nursing, and 2. administrator in the organization. McClure said that people are realizing that patients are admitted to inpatient facilities because they need nursing care. This makes nursing and the nurse executive an important part of the organization's success. The nurse administrator must recognize and develop his/her own potential and that of their followers and be able to see the big picture of the organization. "We must be articulate in helping policymakers to understand that, in hospital care, ultimate responsibility rests with nursing" (p. 7).

Clearly, most authors recognize the need for nurse executives to be connected to nursing and yet participate in the overall organizational directions. What is not so clear in the literature is that the art of caring is the link to the different roles and to their practice as a whole. It seems to be assumed, but not specifically identified as the ability that makes the other abilities work. Without a caring foundation, it seems to me that nursing administration would be a miserable and impossible chore. The stresses between nursing goals and organization goals might pull administrators apart if they could not see that caring is what is needed most in both situations. Caring is what continues the tie of executives to practicing nurses, and it makes the organizational life bearable.

So, where do nursing administrators learn their leadership abilities? Redman (1995) taped the life histories of some chief nurse executives, and they found that fathers were important in many executives' lives. Education was valued, and the executives were often involved in leadership in school, community, or home. These leaders had visionary goals for their organization and the ability to motivate staff to believe their visions. They were open, honest, and personal, empowering to staff, encouraged risk taking, and approached problems from a macro perspective. They showed professional excellence and identified quality patient care as their primary responsibility.

Dunbam et al. (1993) also studied nurse executives. Out of the eighty-five executives, seventeen felt that no person, event, or experience influenced their leadership style. They thought that their leadership abilities were inherent. The rest of the executives, acknowledged that various people, experiences, and events influenced had their leadership styles. In many cases, influential persons had acknowledged and valued them as individuals on both a personal and professional level. This encouraged the nurse executives to expand their views. The conclusion was that leadership abilities are often inherent but further shaping occurs throughout life.

Johnson (1989) examined the power of chief nurse executives (CNEs) and other non-nursing executives with similar titles. She found that the nurses were more powerful in overall normative power, prestige, and esteem, as well as legitimacy of position. They were equal in symbols of power to other administrators. She concludes that nurse executives have a significant impact on the business of health care, and that nurses should cease referring to themselves and their profession as being powerless.

Borman (1993) also CNEs and chief executive officers (CEOs). She found that the CNEs, more than CEOs, could discern, comprehend, visualize, conceptualize, and articulate to their colleagues the opportunities and threats facing their organization. The CNEs had increased scores for flexibility and connection to others, human management knowledge, negotiation/compromise skills, and political savvy. Borman wrote that CNE's skills, styles, and managerial values may benefit women and female executives in emerging organizations.

Stevens (1985) writes that management literature has reflected a basic division between a focus on people and a focus on tasks. Certainly, we have discussed repeatedly that nurses sometimes focus on tasks and sometimes on people. Stevens suggests viewing nursing administration as made up of roles that begin to break down the traditional dichotomy between task and people. She defines a role as something to be put on at the appropriate times and taken off at others. The role and the person are not the same. However, existentialists would disagree because they would say that you are who you are in the roles that you play—a person's essence is in the roles he/she plays. I agree with the existentialists that you cannot play roles that you are not. However, it is sometimes helpful to examine the roles in our lives. Stevens says there are two kinds of roles—ascribed and achieved. Nurse administrators' roles are both achieved (earned) and ascribed (given by authority). She suggests that it is to the executives' advantage to take an aggressive role at the beginning of their job, because it is easier to "back off" later if necessary. I would prefer to take it easier at the beginning of a job so that I can understand the organization before taking strong stands on controversial issues. Stevens describes Mintzberg's ten roles that executives play (it is important to recall that Mintzberg used only males in his study). The roles were: figurehead, leader, liaison, monitor, disseminator, spokesman, entrepreneur, disturbance handler, resource allocator, and negotiator (Mintzberg, 1975). Katz (1974) defines three roles for managers: remediator role (corrective deficiencies and past inefficiencies), maintaining role (preserve a steady balance), and innovative role (start new projects in new directions). While one cannot argue with these roles, they do not include anything about caring for people or intuitive thinking.

Stevens says that it is important for nurse administrators to define and be aware of their own roles (typically related to their special talents) and analyze them critically in light of the needs of the organization. Stevens wrote about the changes in nursing administration in light of new systems where the nurse may become a corporate player. These corporate nurse executives may be in charge of multiple nursing organizations or they may have staff jobs that include advising directors of nursing rather than being able to tell them what to do. These nurse executives need to be able to focus upward and outward with ease, serve as figureheads, have good public-relations skills, and good marketing and strategic planning skills. They serve as role models for the directors of nursing and build corporation-wide systems for nurses.

While role theory has a long history in sociology, it has limitations. The first one is that people get so focused on their roles that they don't pay attention to who they are. Yes, nurse executives must play roles, but they must be very sure of their beliefs and values, and practice from a constant frame of reference. For me, that frame of reference is caring. Nurse executives should play all their roles with caring as the central value.

Another issue concerning nurse administrators is that of mentoring. Holloran (1993) surveyed 274 nurse executives about their experiences with mentoring. She defined a mentor as a more experienced career role model who guides, coaches, and advises the less seasoned person. The mentor has an intensive commitment and strong belief in the potential strengths and talents of the protégé. In mentoring, there are two themes: power of belief; and power of control. The power of belief infuses the protégé with confidence and inspiration. As the mentor shows faith in the protégé, he/she will feel that he/she must be worth the investment. In contrast, the power of control is smothering to the creative aspects of the

A Caring Approach in Nursing Administration

relationship. The mentor may become overpossessive, reject the protégé, or misuse the power in the relationship. The mentor who uses the power of belief encourages, recognizes, and gives opportunities and responsibilities, providing inspiration and helping with career moves. Holloran concludes that mentoring plays a critical role in developing and grooming of nurse leaders. Having a mentor does help one to succeed and to move to a higher organizational position with authority and influence. Nursing administrators should look for mentors and for opportunities to recognize and develop younger members of the nursing profession.

Carey and Campbell (1994) also looked at mentoring and found that mentor relationships have been linked with early career advancement, better education, and improved job satisfaction. Schlotfeld (1985) wrote about the importance of mentoring in developing nurse-scholars. She wrote that mentoring should be sustained, collegial, comfortable, and beneficial to both members of the dyad.

I believe that mentoring can greatly help nurse administrators in their careers. I had a mentor whom I met in graduate school, and she helped me in many aspects of my career. I also looked for others to mentor. I had graduate students work with me and I encouraged many potential leaders to return to school or pursue career moves. To me, mentoring was a part of being caring. It provided opportunities for me to share myself with others, and I still keep in touch with my mentor and those I have mentored. They are special relationships to me.

Another issue is that of practicing nursing administration from a theoretical framework. DiVencenti (1989) says that the practice of nursing administration needs to be symbiotic in relation to theory and inquiry. "Use of theory enables nurse administrators to make clearer sense of complex situations and to formulate the best possible strategies for rational action. Without a strong grounding in the finest knowledge, we run the risk of floundering aimlessly at work in a random tide" (p. 567).

Meleis and Jennings (1989) also wrote that nursing administration has not attended to nursing theory as fundamental to its scientific growth. Theory is also a coherent, communicable articulation and conceptualization of responses to health and illness by human beings in their environments. Theory is a cyclical, ongoing process that is based on philosophical premises, practice patterns, results of research, scientific statements, and experience and history. Meleis and Jennings think that the current practice of nursing administration is guided primarily by theories in the business world. They call for a joining of knowledge of management and nursing to blend, transform, and balance the two sources of knowledge. They believe that bridges can be built to connect theories and form a synthesis of a nursing perspective with organizational, financial, psychological, and sociological theories that are relevant to nursing. These authors agree with Blair that education for nursing administration has lagged behind other nursing specialties, and that has resulted in nurses getting their graduate education in business schools. This may promote one's allegiance with management at the expense of nursing. Nursing leaders need advanced education in nursing theories and research to be leaders of a caring nursing discipline. Nursing administrators are responsible for the development of a nursing culture (values, norms, sanctions, rewards, and behaviors that are shared by a group of people) that is based on caring and a focus on patient care. Nursing administration is perceived negatively by some nurses, and using nursing theories in administrative systems may reduce those feelings.

This book is based on a nursing theory—the theory of caring. But instead of just reiterating the caring theory, I have tried to make a theoretical framework for nursing administration—caring nursing administration. We have started with the concept of caring and delineated a basis, understanding, and application to make caring realized in nursing administration. This is an attempt to begin to identify theories of nursing administration based on nursing theories, but infused into nursing administration by application of the caring precepts into all areas of nursing administration. It is an attempt at theory building for a specialized part of nursing—nursing administration.

The theory of caring administration refers us back to the beginning assumptions in this book. Now, we must practice the assumptions:

1. We treat people as integrated, whole individuals, and we do not try to understand them piece by piece. We set up systems that honor the holism of patients and of nurses. We understand the organization as a whole and do our part to diminish competition and encourage harmony toward organizational goals.

2. We see health and illness as a dynamic, fluctuating continuum in the health care system. Health is a state of harmony of body, mind, and spirit, and caring administration continuously seeks health for patients/families, nurses, and the organization.

3. Nursing is a caring, holistic relationship between the nurse and patient. Nursing is also caring relationships with all nurses and with others who make up our work world. I believe we can nurse the organization by empowering employees and developing the theme of caring throughout the organization.

4. The environment is viewed as an integral unit in which caring relationships take place. The environment may be the patient's room, or it may be all societal milieus. The caring nursing administrator understands the importance of a calming, caring environment that enhances growth for all involved.

5. Nursing administration is a specialized practice of nursing that includes elements of caring and sharing, financial and managerial knowledge, ethical foundations, and systems development. It uses knowledge and skills of management, nursing, and caring in its practice.

6. Nursing administrative practice is creating, monitoring, and evaluating systems for nursing practice. It is greatly influenced by underlying values and beliefs. The central value is caring, and the nurse administrator must believe that nurses share caring values and beliefs about holistic patient care. The values and beliefs of caring are the cornerstone of nursing administration practice.

7. Nursing administrators develop a work environment that is caring and encourages autonomy and creativity. Power is shared power as nurses seek collegial relationships throughout the organization. When contemplating changes in structures, the caring nursing administrator must ask how they will contribute to the caring goal.

As we review the assumptions, it is clear that the way nursing administrators care is most often related to caring for nurses and caring for the organization. We devise structures and systems and treat everyone in a way that encourages organizational caring. We are equal participants in organizational management and remain the leaders of a caring profession.

We can reiterate from the first chapter that caring can permeate our thinking about organizations and it can change the way we practice nursing administration. The material in this book has been chosen to be useful to nurse administrators who wish to make caring central to their work.

We are reminded that caring is relationships and it is growth. It involves ways of behaving toward other people. It makes a difference in our priorities and gives life greater meaning. It is a natural and fulfilling part of practicing nursing and practicing nursing administration.

A few years ago, I taught a class about caring nursing administration. At the end of the class, the students and I put together a list of attributes that we believed are highly developed in caring nurse administrators. Some of the attributes can be found in many "good" managers, but we believed the attributes were more highly developed in caring administrators. The attributes are:

1. *Philosophy of caring.* Caring as a philosophy is a conscious goal for these administrators. The philosophy permeates their every action; not just in nursing, but the whole constellation of their behaviors.

2. *Fairness.* This is an attribute that may be found among many administrators, but the caring administrator recognizes the potential of all the people around them. They are acutely aware that fairness is a must if caring is being demonstrated.

3. *Professionalism.* The caring administrator sees his/her commitment to nursing as a lifelong affair. It is not a job, it is a calling, and there is a knowledge base that goes with being a professional. Nursing is a profession of dignity and compassion that stays with the professional all the time, not just at work. A nurse is always a nurse, and he/she responds to daily life from this point of view.

4. *Craftsman.* As we have seen in this book, there are different ways to organize nursing's work. But the nurse desires the work that contributes clearly to the well-being of the patient. It is unprofessional and uncaring to divide nurses' work into tasks that have no relation to the patient outcome. The nurse is a craftsperson in caring/healing, and being able to deal repeatedly and continuously with the patient is the only way for them to practice their profession.

5. *Collegiality.* The caring nurse administrator treats all nurses with the respect of colleagues. The more we can encourage organizations that allow nurses ultimate patient care decisions and direct input into organizational affairs, the more nurses can feel like colleagues. Caring administrators do not feel like they need power for themselves, but are interested in all nurses reaching their full potential.

6. *Planning and creativity.* The caring administrator plans for the future of nursing and the organization, allows nurses to show creativity in their work, and encourages their input into organizational matters. Activities done helter-skelter do not show that a person cares about the activities of their work. Creativity shows respect for all persons in the organization, and helps the organization meet new challenges head-on.

7. *Power as influence.* Caring administrators spread power, not hoard it. They feel secure in their own use of power, but do not feel the need to use power to gain compliance to their wishes. Power is an opportunity, not a battle cry. It is something to be used carefully to enhance nursing and the organization.

8. *Open communication and decision making.* This may be the most important attribute of the caring administrator. Open communication means being able to listen to good and bad information. It means you have to be accessible to people so they can communicate with you. It means asking for clarification, not cutting communication off when things get hot. It includes letting people in on the problems and the accolades, and letting others participate in decision making. Mostly, it means sharing—yourself and your work so that as many people as possible feel like a part of things.

9. *Fiscal accountability.* As much as we get frustrated about finances, it is ultimately caring to practice fiscal accountability. Resources are limited and everybody tries to get as big a piece of the pie as possible. But the caring administrator uses resources as efficiently as possible and encourages others to do the same. I have expressed my view that sharing responsibility for finances with nurses is a wise and effective measure of control. I believe that if we make finances a little less ominous and quit using them as a fear tactic, teamwork could emerge and make financial accountability a real possibility.

10. *Environment of excellence.* Caring nurse administrators expect a lot, not a little, when it comes to the work of patient care. Expecting excellence shows respect for nurses by saying, "I know you can do it well." Equally important is the recognition of excellent work. Caring means encouraging people to do their work well and feeling

good about it. The storytelling technique mentioned earlier struck me as an excellent way for nurses to share their work with administrators in a meaningful way.

11. *Management by relationships.* I believe that this attribute is one that probably cannot be done by a noncaring administrator. Nurses' work with patients is, most of all, relationship-oriented, and this ability makes it possible for nurse administrators to extend the caring of relationships into administration. The relationship technique means talking things over with people. It means asking instead of telling. It means being in full attendance at every conversation. It means hearing not just words, but meanings. It means people work with you, not for you, and that is the crux of caring administration.

12. *Autonomy, potential, and empowerment of staff.* The caring administrator believes that people work better when they are treated as if they are very important. Sometimes it is easier to do the work yourself than to delegate it, but caring means trusting that people have potential which can be achieved in an empowering environment. It means not looking over someone's shoulder as they make decisions, but trusting them to make the right decision on their own.

13. *Altruistic values.* The caring administrator believes in the innate good of people and is willing to help others just for the reward of doing so. They give of themselves to others and encourage others to do the same. Caring *is* giving.

14. *Integrity and personal excellence.* Caring administrators expects a lot of others, but no more than they expect of themselves. They do their work completely, comprehensively, and as well as they can. They have high moral and ethical values that they incorporate into all of their lives. The very act of caring depends on personal integrity and excellence.

I believe that caring nurse administrators have great respect for nursing at all levels. They recognize their responsibility to care for nurses as they expect nurses to care for patients. They remain available to nurses and recognize their two primary roles: 1. being a leader of a caring profession, and 2. being a facilitator of caring in the health care organization. They use their time wisely, delegating when possible (even recognizing that sometimes asking a busy person is the best way to get things done), and realizing that they and the nurses have to have a healthy life outside of their work. Life must be seen in its totality, and caring is the foundation for a healthy life.

When someone writes a book, they try to cover all the bases—to have answers for everything. I do not feel that way about this book. I see it as the beginning of an understanding of the uniqueness of nursing administration. I have tried to lay a sound foundation to justify extended study and exploration about the ideal of a new kind of nurse administrator—a caring nursing administrator.

I end this book by recognizing two more points about the work of the caring nurse administrator. The first point I want to make is that no nursing administrator has the information to do a perfect job. Etzioni (1989) wrote about humble decision making. He said that executives in our modern era must often proceed with only partial information that they have no time to fully process or analyze. In simpler ages, decisions were held to be made rationally after exploring every route and collecting complete information about the costs and utility of each alternative. For today's executive, this is not feasible. At best we can gather limited information, allowing our intuitive self to learn and understand as much as possible. Etzioni suggests that executives take part in information gathering, recognizing the incompleteness of the data. The data is scanned and consideration is given to a broad range of facts and choices. Incremental decisions are then made and evaluated at intervals to check progress toward the goals. Commitment to revise course as necessary is maintained and information continues to be gathered. Essential qualities of today's executives are maintaining flexibility, caution, and the capacity to proceed with partial knowledge.

I find this perspective to be important for all executives, but particularly for nursing administrators. If you have to know all the information before proceeding with things, not much will get done in today's information-overloaded systems. It seems to me that caring nursing administrators will be in a better place to proceed with business if they do not expect to do the job alone. Inclusive management means letting others into the process, and that is what the caring nurse administrator will do by nature of the caring. The organization will be open, flexible, and creative as all nursing professionals join the process of management.

In speaking to a vice president of nursing at a local hospital, I found that she also emphasizes the importance of working with people and being flexible. She feels that the ability to get people to work together in a multidisciplinary manner will be the key to developing creative patient care systems that put the patient first, and these systems are key to health care's future. We need to get nurses to work together and then bring all care providers into these systems where everyone can feel good about what they bring to patient care outcomes. Nurses and nurse administrators must be more than flexible—they must be *improvisational* in getting old stuff together in new ways that focus on caring for patients.

The last point I want to make comes from Bateson's 1990 book, *Composing a Life.* She says that the old model of success was for a person to make early decisions and commitments to live their lives in a single trajectory (like becoming a nurse). But now our lives not only take new directions, they are subject to repeated redirection. We must learn the art of improvisation by recombining partly familiar materials in new ways. It is time to explore our creative potential, where energies are not narrowly focused or permanently pointed toward a single ambition. We must view life as a patchwork of achievements, both personally and professionally, and we must look at how they fit together to "compose a life." Our utmost need is to sustain human growth and compose a life that involves an openness to possibilities and the capacity to put them together in a way that they fit like patches in a patchwork quilt. "The real winners in a rapidly changing world will be those who are open to alternatives and able to respect and value those who are different" (p. 74). These thoughts are things that I have had to implement in my life as I faced a disability that ended my career as a nursing administrator. But other parts of life have opened up for me, and I no longer spend tremendous amounts of energy trying to regain what is gone. For example, I would never have had the time or concentration to write this book if I were still a practicing nursing administrator. Nurse administrators can be very committed to their jobs, and then suddenly find themselves out of work. Or, even in their work things can change so drastically that changes must occur in their lives. I think that a caring nursing administrator has a better handle on reacting to change because she knows that wherever she goes and no matter what the change, caring will go with her and sustain her. Life in general and life in organizations are indeed like patchwork quilts, and whatever we do and

A Caring Approach in Nursing Administration

wherever we go, we can make meaning in our lives as long as caring is our guiding principle. We will compose our lives in various situations and various missions, and, at the end, we will have the satisfaction of knowing that we did our caring work well.

References

Bateson, M. C. (1990). *Composing a Life*. New York: A Plume Book.

Blair, E. M. (1976). Needed—nursing administration leaders. *Nursing Outlook* 27 (9): 550–554.

———. (1989). Nursing and administration: A synthesis model. *Nursing Administration Quarterly* 13 (2): 1–11.

Borman, J. C. (1993). Women and nurse executives: Finally, some advantages. *The Journal of Nursing Administration* 23 (10): 34–41.

Carey, S. J. and S. T. Campbell (1994). Preceptor, mentor, and sponsor roles: Creative strategies for nurse retention. *The Journal of Nursing Administration* 24 (2): 39–48.

DiVencenti, M. (1989). Introduction: The practice of nursing administration. In B. Henry, C. Arndt, M. DiVencenti, and A. Marriner-Tomey, eds., *Dimensions of Nursing Administration*. Boston: Blackwell Scientific Publications, pp. 567–569.

Dunbam, J., F. Taylor, E. Fisher, and E. Kinion (1993). Experiences, events, people: Do they influence the leadership style of nurse executives. *The Journal of Nursing Administration* 23 (7–8): 30–34.

Etzioni, A. (1989). Humble decision making. *Harvard Business Review* 67 (4): 122–126.

Holloran, S. D. (1993). Mentoring: The experiences of nursing service executives. *The Journal of Nursing Administration* 23 (2): 49–54.

Johnson P. T. (1989). The normative power of chief executive nurses. *Image: Journal of Nursing Scholarship* 21 (3): 162–167.

Katz, R. L. (1974). Skills of an effective administrator. *Harvard Business Review* 52 (5): 91–92.

Klakovich, M. D. (1994). Connective leadership for the 21st century: A historical perspective and future direction. *Advances in Nursing Science* 16 (4): 42–54.

McClure, M. L. (1989). The nurse executive role: A leadership opportunity. *Nursing Administration Quarterly* 13 (3): 1–8.

Meleis, A. I. and B. M. Jennings (1989). Theoretical nursing administration: Today's challenges, tomorrow's bridges. In C. Arndt, M. DiVencenti, and A. Marriner-Tomey, eds., *Dimensions of Nursing Administration*. Boston: Blackwell Scientific Publications, pp. 7–17.

Miller, K. L. (1989). Nurse executive leadership: A corporate perspective. *Nursing Administration Quarterly* 13 (2): 12–18.

Mintzberg, H. (1975). The manager's job: Folklore and fact. *Harvard Business Review* 53 (4): 49–61.

Redman, G. M. (1995). We don't make widgets here: Voices of chief executive nurses. *The Journal of Nursing Administration* 25 (2): 63–69.

Sarosi, G. M. and P. O. O'Conner (1993). The microstory pathway of executive nursing rounds: Tales of living caring. *Nursing Administration Quarterly* 16 (4): 1–8.

Schlotfield, R. (1985). Mentorship: A means to desirable ends. In J. C. McCloskey and H. K. Grace, eds., *Current Issues in Nursing*. Boston: Blackwell Scientific Publications.

Schoenhofer, L. O. (1994). Transforming visions for nursing in the time world of Einstein's dreams. *Advances in Nursing Science* 13 (2): 1–11.

Smith, P. M., R. J. Parsons, B. P. Murray, R. M. Dwors, and V. M. Vorderer (1994). The new nurse executive: An emerging role. *The Journal of Nursing Administration* 24 (11): 56–62.

Stevens, B. J. (1985). *The Nurse as Executive*. Rockville, MD: Aspen Publications.

Stivers, C. (1991). Why can't a women be less like a man? *The Journal of Nursing Administration* 21 (5): 47–51.

Index

Care: enhancing, 52–53, 140, 205; evaluation of, 215; lack of, 219; maintaining, 178, 182; quality, 52, 157, 199, 206; relationship-centered, 19, 189. *See also* Health care

Care delivery systems, 171; changing, 213

Career ladders, 69, 211; working on, 212

Carefoote, R.: on TQM, 201, 202

Care pairs, 52, 53

Care Q, 177; development of, 178; using, 175, 179, 181

Care/Sat questionnaire, 177, 178, 185

Carey, S. J.: on mentoring, 239

Caring, 1, 84, 116, 151, 162, 200, 202, 233; bureaucratic, 24, 176, 185; components of, 14, 15, 16, 29, 30–37, 177; concept of, 10, 18, 25; defining, 27, 36, 175; facilitator of, 6; focusing on, 19, 32; as foundational, 229; healthy life and, 245; human dignity and, 13; implementing, 98, 189; increasing, 24, 55, 118; as individuality, 17, 158; as interacting, 18; as knowing, 17; meaning of, 36–37; mentoring, 239; models for, 206; organizational, 241; philosophy of, 188, 189, 209, 242; practices of, 16–17; as presence, 17; therapeutic part of, 21

Caring (Noddings), 153

Caring Assessment Scale, 186, 189; development of, 178; sample of, 180

Caring Behaviors Inventory (CBI), 173, 177, 185, 186; development of, 178

Caring ethic, 28, 60, 153, 154, 155, 162, 228; constraints on, 130

Caring modalities, teaching, 188–89

Caring theory, 3, 5, 6, 45, 53, 73, 240–41; organization theory and, 43–44

"Carrier bag" theory, 218

Case management, 63, 112, 140, 170, 206, 211, 216–17; nursing and, 113

Case mix, reducing, 216

CBI. *See* Caring Behaviors Inventory

CEOs. *See* Chief executive officers

Change: organizational, 42, 184–85; propensity for, 63; significant, 222

Chief executive officers (CEOs), 237

Chief nurse executives (CNEs), 237; leadership abilities of, 236

Childress, J. F.: on ethics committees, 152

Cleland, V. S.: on economics, 122, 132; on health care needs/wants, 131; on nurses, 137, 139; on productivity, 138; on salaries, 137

Clinical nurses, 112, 223, 230

Clinical studies, 210; variables affecting, 170

Clinton, Bill: health care and, 106, 107, 108, 109

Clinton, Hillary: on nurses/health care, 111

CNEs. *See* Chief nurse executives

Collaborators: followership and, 222–23; leaders and, 222, 223

Collegiality, 78, 152, 230, 242

Columbus, Christopher: paradigm change and, 74

Comforting, 173, 176, 178

Commitment, 36, 179, 184, 230, 245, 246; caring and, 30; emotional, 81; fostering, 165; success and, 201; value, 81

Communication, 36, 160, 176; caring and, 19, 20, 30; meaning and, 71; open, 243; organizations and, 39

Competency, 79, 143

Competent nurse, described, 210

Competition, 58, 106, 132; cooperation and, 204; monopoly and, 129

Composing a Life (Bateson), 246

Conglomerates, 51, 158

Conjoint professional organization, 226; described, 225

Connectedness, 45, 53, 198, 232–33; autonomy and, 218; caring and, 28; value of, 145

Consumer sovereignty, 122, 123, 159, 202

Contextual variables, 171, 186–87, 189

Contingency theory, 46

Continuity, 172, 202

Control, 97, 221; professional/administrative zones of, 224

Cooper, M. C.: on ethics, 153

Cooperation, 56, 58, 187; competition and, 204

Coordination, 39, 229

Cost-benefit analysis, 130, 132

Costs, 93, 100, 106, 108, 195; administrative, 113, 124; care and, 203; containing, 75, 94, 95, 97–99, 101–03, 109, 113–15, 123, 126, 139, 162; excessive, 96; increase in, 95, 126, 129, 130; outcomes and, 97; prioritizing, 92; problems with, 131; quality and, 123. *See also* Prices

Covenantal ethics, 160, 161–62

Covey, S. R., 74; caring theory and, 73; on human motivation, 72; on ineffective people, 72; on principle-centered leaders, 72–73; on TQM, 73

Craftsman, 242

Creative Nursing Administration: Participative Management into the 21st Century (Porter-O'Grady), 63–64

Creative Nursing Management (Porter-O'Grady), 67

Creativity, 53, 70, 233; conflict and, 198; planning and, 243

Cronin, S. N.: on nursing research, 164

Culture, 81; caring and, 15–16; corporate, 235; leadership-oriented, 61; masculine, 234; nursing, 240; service-oriented, 200

Current theoretic organizations, types of, 66

Curtin, L. L.: on ethics, 162; on medical diagnoses, 217; on transformational leadership, 85

D

Davis, G.: on nursing/health policy, 111

Decision making, 243, 245

Delegation, 35, 70

Demand, need vs., 134

Deming, W. Edwards, 205; on managers, 204; on organizations, 56, 58, 204; on suppliers, 223

Diagnostic related groupings (DRGs), 13, 102, 123, 128, 130, 217

DiVencenti, M.: on theory, 239

Dix, Dorothea: nursing reform and, x

"Do good" rule, 153

Doing for, 17

Donabedian, A.: on commitment/accountability, 184

Donahue, M. P., ix

"Do no harm" principle, 152

DRGs. *See* Diagnosis-related groupings

Dunbam, J.: on nurse executives, 236–37

Dzurec, L. C.: on quantitative studies, 166; on science, 166–67

E

Economics, 5; caring and, 13, 24–25, 122, 129, 131, 132, 140, 141, 142, 179, 183, 184; complexity of, 130; human care and, 181, 183–84, 185; normative, 122; nurses and, 121, 131, 136, 139–40; questions about, 182, 186; understanding, 122, 127, 139–40. *See also* Budgeting

Eddy, D.: on control mechanisms, 97; on physicians/health care market, 96

Education, 211, 231, 240; caring, 188; programs for, 58

Edwards, P. A.: on health care industry, 214

Edwards, R.: on nurse managers, 82

Effective followers, developing, 80

Effectiveness, 82, 202; measuring, 193, 195; organizational, 83, 193–96

Efficiency, 202; improvements in, 158; organizations and, 40; pursuit of, 161

"Element of Caring in Nursing Administration, The" (Gaut and Mayeroff), 185

Ellsworth, R. R.: on integrity, 61; on leadership, 85, 150; on managers, 61–62

Employees: fundamental needs of, 221; satisfaction of, 194; training, 41; treatment of, 157, 205

Employers: insurance and, 99–100, 103; managed care and, 100, 104

Empowerment, 160, 241, 244

Enabling, 17

Entrepreneurship, autonomy and, 50

Environment, 4, 8, 241

Erickson, E. H., 145; on nursing administration, xi; on student nurses, 14–15

Estes, C.: on costs, 107; on health care policy, 93

Ethics, viii, 5, 14, 151, 158, 241; articulating, 161; bad, 161, 198; business, 156, 157, 160, 162; caring, 28, 130, 153, 154, 155, 162, 228; covenantal, 160, 161–62; egalitarian, 91; importance of, 152, 162; marketing, 159; principle-centered, 153; survival, 160; thinking about, 144; values and, 156, 157, 158; women and, 149, 154

Ethics committees, 152, 153

Etzioni, A.: on decision making, 245

Excellence, 74, 243–44

Expert nurses: described, 210; instructions by, 210–11

F

Facilitators, 63, 232, 244; caring and, 6, 178; role of, 235

Fagin, C. M.: on nurse-doctor game, 111

Fairness, 81, 152, 242

Farrell, T.: on deep values, 84; on leadership/connectiveness, 84

Female Advantage: Women's Ways of Leading, The (Helgesen), 147

Feminism, 136, 234. *See also* Women

Ferhetich, S. F.: on caring, 177

Fifth discipline, 59–60

Fifth Discipline, The (Senge), 58

Financing, 91, 98, 217, 241

Fitzpatrick, M. J.: on procedures/performance, 202

Flexibility, importance of, 246

Focus groups, 187–88

Followership, 79–80; collaborators and, 222–23

Foster, R.: on normative economics, 122

Freedom, restraints on, 183

Freel, M. I.: on truth-telling, 154, 155

Free-market competition system, 128, 129

Freud, Sigmund, 145

Friedman, E.: on health care inequities, 115

From Novice to Expert (Benner), 21, 205, 209

Fuchs, V. C.: on ethics/health care, 91

Fun, big/little, 83–84

G

Gaut, D., 185; on caring, 11, 29

Gillem, T. R.: on hospitals/Deming's theory, 56–57

Gilligan, Carol, 144, 146

Gilman, M. P.: on research, 170

Gilmore, Anna: on managed care, 114

Ginzberg, E.: on health care reform, 108

Goals, 156, 194–95; attaining, 193; defining, 58; nursing/ administration, 236

Goode, C. J.: on process/outcome, 203; on research, 169

Governance models, 223; shared, 67, 221, 226; self-, 211, 221–22, 226

Greeneich, D., 200; on business/quality care, 199

Growth, 182, 246; caring and, 11, 36, 37, 242

H

Haas, S. A.: on research, 169

Habits of the Heart (Bellah), 135

Hailstones, T. J.: on economics, 122, 132

Harrington, C.: on nurses/health care reform, 110

Havens, D. C.: on shared governance, 221

Havens, D. S.: on work structures/ effectiveness, 82

Hawthorn studies, 43–44

Hayne, A. N.: on power/leadership, 79

Healing, 82; caring and, 20; responsibility for, 28

Health: described, 4; determinants of, 96; illness and, 240; pollutants/lifestyle and, 96

Health care: as business, 90, 98; caring in, 65, 89, 97, 115; changes in, 8, 65, 75, 90; government influence in, 93, 105–6; interpretation of, 7–8; needs/wants in, 131; priority for, 134; problems for, 90, 95, 99, 106–7; spending on, 92–93, 99. *See also* Care

"Health Care Economics and Human Caring in Nursing; Why the Moral Conflict Must Be Resolved" (Ray), 24

Healthcare Forum Journal, 52

Health care reform, 103, 104, 107–8, 109; caring and, 17; debate over, 93, 112, 217; needs/demands and, 134; nurses and, xii, 110, 111–12, 214

Health care system, 6, 93; caring and, 89, 115; changes in, 65, 89, 106; criticism of, 116; oligopolistic, 129

Health maintenance organizations (HMOs), 94, 159; cost cutting by, 102, 103–4; employers and, 100, 104; insurance companies and, 100; managed care and, 99; merging of, 101; physician practices and, 158; problems with, 100–101, 102, 103, 104; strategy of, 100

Joint Commission of Accreditation of Health Care Organizations (JCAHO), 42, 202

Jones, C. B.: on technology/caring, 141–42

Journal of Nursing Administration, 85, 178

Judgments, 145, 176

K

Kaiser Permanente, 100

Kantor, R.: on bosses/subordinates, 80; on success, 53, 80–81; on work structures/effectiveness, 82

Katz, R. L.: on management roles, 238

Keirsey, D.: on personality types, 86

Kellogg Foundation, 230

Kevorkian, Jack, 133, 152

Kingry, M. J.: on focus groups, 188

Klakovich, M. D.: on abandonment, 232; on leadership, 235

Knafl, K. A.: on confirmation, 167

Knowing, 16

Kohlberg, 145; on ethics, 151

Kotter, J. P.: on leadership, 60–61, 70, 71; on managers, 69

Kramer, M.: Magnet Hospital study and, 51

Kuhn, T.: on paradigms, 8

L

Lamm, Richard: rationing and, 92

Larson, E.: on outcomes/quality, 172, 203

Larson, P. J.: Care Q and, 175; Care/Sat and, 185; caring and, 11, 175, 177

Laschinger, H. K. S.: on work structures/effectiveness, 82

Lathrop, J. Philip, 52

Lawton, B. B.: on Deming's philosophy, 56

Leaders, 78, 232, 238, 244; advice for, 77; collaborators and, 222, 223; developing/grooming, 239; education for, 240; human skills of, 71; values-driven, 62

Leadership, 6, 80, 83, 84; connective, 235; effective, 71; female, 49, 234; management and, 71, 83; movement and, 60; nursing administration and, 69; paradigms of, 222, 224; people-centered, 72–73; potential for, 228–30; power in, 79; principle-centered, 72; responsibility of, 62; style of, viii, 85, 236–37; system improvement and, 57; transactional, 85; transformational, 71, 85; types of, 62–63, 84, 85; vision/voice and, 148

Leadership and the Quest for Integrity (Badarocco and Ellsworth), 61

Learning, 59; importance of, 70, 72

Lee, P. R.: on costs, 106, 108; on health care policy, 93

Leininger, M.: on caring, 11, 29

Leisure: altruism vs., 135–36; focus on, 136

Levinson, H.: on art of caring, 97

Liberation Management (Peters), 51

Life, importance of, 133

Likert, on management systems, 44, 45

Listening, 161, 173; intuitive, 232–33

Litigation, fear of, 109, 136

Litman, T. J.: on change, 106; on federalism, 105

Living wills, 133

Locke, John: on freedom/security, 183

Lodahl, T. M.: on positive maturity, 55

Megatrends, emergence of, 48–49

Megatrends (Naisbitt), 48

Megatrends for Women, 149

Megatrends 2000 (Naisbitt and Aburdene), 48

Megel, M. E.: on QA/QI nurse professionals, 198

Meleis, A. I.: on administration theory, 239–40

Mentoring, 238–39

Merriner-Tomey, A.: on organizing, 39

Mersmann, C. A.: on research, 170

Metanoia, 59

Metaparadigm, 168, 222

Miller, K. L.: on clinical studies, 170; on contextual variables, 171; on facilitators, 235; on nurse administrators/caring, 22, 30, 168–69

Mintzberg, H.: on executive roles, 238; on male managers, 147

Mitchell, S. M.: on positive maturity, 55

Money: donating, 136; emphasis on, 182

Monopoly system, 128, 129

Montgomery, C. L.: on caring, 19, 20

Morale, 220

Morality, 145, 209

Moral mazes, 156, 157

Morgan, C. P.: on organizational effectiveness, 195

Morgan, Gareth: on bureaucracy, 53; on imaginization, 54; on imposition of rules, 39; organization metaphors by, 53–54, 55; on systems approach, 45; on work responsibilities, 53

Morse, J. M.: on work patterns, 212–13

Motivation, 35–36, 161

Murphy, D.: on nurses/followers, 79–80

N

Naisbitt, James: on management, 48

Nanus, R.: on leadership, 71, 77

Nash, L.: on business ethics, 160, 162; on covenantal ethics, 160, 161–62

National health board, 107, 109

Naval Air Systems Command, TQM and, 201

Naylor, M.: on patient outcomes, 171

Need, demand vs., 134

Net revenue expectation, 124

Newborns, caring and, 174–75

Nightingale, Florence, 28, 171

Nixon, Richard: HMOs and, 100

Noddings, N., 185; on caring, 10, 28, 32; on ethics, 153–54; on openness, 34

Noncoercive influence strategies, 222

Non-nurses, 187, 216

Novice nurses, 21; described, 209–10; training, 211

Nugent, P. S.: on managerial modes of thought, 149

Nurse administrators: caring and, 18, 22–23, 25, 29, 30, 31, 33, 36, 65, 159, 168, 216, 231–32, 233, 234, 236, 241, 242–44, 246–47; as clinical experts, 233–34; commitment by, 246; communication by, 36; cost unconsciousness of, 124; delegation by, 35; ethics and, 155, 156, 159, 162–63; goals by, 131; influence of, 78, 159, 200; managing and, 151; organizations and, 47, 184; performance and, 211; personal needs and, 31; planning by, 32, 219; relationships with, 32; reputation of, xi, 78; role of, 235–36, 237, 238; self-worth and, 31; shortage of, 230; staff and, 184, 233, 234, 236; work of, xi, 1, 2, 5, 70, 83–84

Nurse analysts, health care issues and, 112

Nurse entrepreneurs, encouraging, 111

Nurse managers, 22, 67, 197; acknowledging, 35; caring and, 87; potential, 228–30; skills of, 82–83; work/satisfaction and, 82

Nurses: caring and, 12, 13, 18–19, 21, 22, 29, 61, 115–16, 177, 215, 227; caring for, 233, 236, 244; classification of, 209–10; HMOs and, 102; leadership and, 228–30, 232; management and, 75; organization by, xii; patients and, 36, 78, 90, 116, 139, 177, 199–200, 214, 217; shortage of, 137, 179, 219

Nurses' aides, 116, 170, 215; using, 216, 219

Nursing: bureaucracy and, 40, 47, 64; devaluation of, 146; economics of, 121; essence of, 4, 11, 21, 213; health care reform and, 110, 111–12, 214; organizations and, 42; paradigm shifts in, 75; practice/organization of, 208; primary, 211, 214; progression of, xi–xii, 12–13; research and, 172; styles of, 78; technology and, 172

Nursing administration, viii, ix–xii, 4; caring and, ix, 27, 184, 227, 228, 241, 245; caring theory for, 5, 6; commitment by, 230; education for, 240; leadership and, 69; mission of, xi; research on, 164, 167–69, 170; successful, 230; uniqueness of, 245

Nursing administrative practice, described, 4

Nursing shift supervisors, 234

Nursing theory, 140, 141, 165, 239–40; power and, 79

Nuttal, G.: on deep values, 84; on leadership/connectiveness, 84

Nyberg Caring Assessment Scale, 186, 189; development of, 178; sample of, 180

O

O'Conner, P. O.: on connections, 232; on listening, 232–33

O'Malley, O. O.: on research, 169

Openness, 36, 54; caring and, 33–34

Open systems, 54, 194

Operating budget, 125

Organizational drift, 55

Organizational literature, 47–48, 67; conclusions from, 65

Organizational metaphors, 54

Organizational models, 224–26; types of, 224

Organizational structure, 47, 52, 186; changes in, 184–85; technical methods and, 45

Organizational theory, viii, 5, 9, 38, 47, 55–56, 69, 95, 140, 141; caring theory and, 43–44; chart for, 66

Organizations: assessing, 183; beginnings of, 38–39; bureaucratic, 66, 67; care and, 66, 84, 158, 176–77, 203, 241; complex of, 45; controlling, 224–25; current theoretic, 66; economists in, 123; environmental variables and, 8; formal/informal, 39; for-profit, 94, 125, 158; goals of, 58, 194–95; health care, 42, 94, 95; individual freedom and, 183; learning, 59; as machines, 53; matrix, 46; maturation of, 55; not-for-profit,